Unveiling The Pure Healing

Alternative medicine guide to share on the way

RUSIANE ALMEIDA

Printed in the United States of America First Printing, 2020
ISBN 978-1-64826-442-9

Rusiane Almeida
1065 SW 8th ST Unit 313
Miami, FL, 33130
Rusianealmeida@protonmail.com
Rusianealmeida.com

Dedications

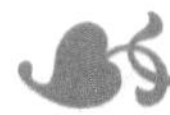

This book is my gift to the world, I am giving back with appreciation for all the blessings the universe allowed me to have in this lifetime and many cycles that has been allowed , I am dedicating to every single one, many ways to touch people's lives positively, Thank you universe, I am years light grateful.

The unconditional love beyond of this reality for my family, Rebecca Quiara and Elisa Mayara, My girls that inspire and guided me to embrace the holistic life, living alternative medicine, overcoming obstacles create a better lifestyle. Love is patient, love is kind, It doe not envy, It does not boast, it is not proud. Thank you for the truth love experience.

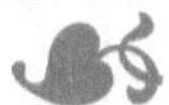

In memory of Dr. Brad Timph chiropractor thank you for continue enlightening many students through dimensions, the support of professor Ms. Linda and Mr. Conrad Timph, I have infinite appreciation for all the kindness that I've received from this beautiful family, the encouragement of Ms. Lee with grace and sweetness of heart and the talented occupational therapist Ms. Abby Timph always guiding people with alternative methods. I am forever thankful for the support, Timph family helped me to recreate and heal in such unique way, wishes of healing for this special family, I am forever thankful.

In memory of Mr. Bohlke II, You thought me that anyone can pursuit a better life with values, share wisely with different culture, you mastered the art of the sea with bravery, we hold you dearly and your researches, your charisma and your love, you will always be reminded through generations, living soulfully, positively changing people's lives, You're your grandchildren's hero, The navy one that honored me the last dance, Thank you Dad I am indeed honored.

In memory of Mr. Almeida my adoptive father that thought me life and in memory sympathy of my brother and love, your help transformed me positively, thank you Dad for your teachings, genuine forgiveness towards the light for my dear brother, The creator, however turned the curse into a blessing. Life is a rare gift, appreciation is everything. Thank you for the precious gift of life.

My gratitude for the ones that directly and indirectly contributed towards this book to become reality, we definitely share common goals as well continue our support for our holistic community.
Thank you Mr. Brian Tracy, Your lecture motivated the manifestation this book, it's possible, you have the art to create positive results, you're pure light. My admiration for your work and family , tremendous magic that you share with the world, it is powerful, Thank you.

My special love for the holistic community in Colorado and Florida, the culture we shared towards health and natural healing supporting the healthy lifestyle and quality of life of people, without this support Amazon Pure Healing would never be possible. Thank you.

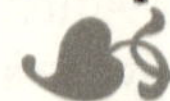

Mr. Bill your help tremendously inspired this book, you showed me alternative ways to create a new reality, you're a mentor thank you for sharing love and the master mind, lighthouse support in moments of healing.
Livia Caudell, Thank you for the motivation and share the holistic values, the generation of healers, absolutely magical, Thank you soul sister.
Ms. Nair Sobrinho back to the roots of the amazon healing, you're a mother, thank you, you thought me the complexities of natural healing, you helped me translate this language with a simple approach, my sincere admiration, with high regards for the Amazon Healers.
My sincere admiration for the ones that practice the holistic living with body, mind and soul, Mr. Steven your courage manifested miracles, your story inspired me and proved that beyond any theory the power of believe, nature and surrender is a gift from the creator. Thank you for Sharing light.
Dr. Ricci female soul, from the day you crossed my path, I was finishing this study, it has been a pleasure share the beautiful holistic living on the virtues and the real meaning of practicing alternative healing, thank you for your wisdom, the moments with nature, you showed me Sincere holistic healing and nature.
Thank you Dr. Jeremy Grantham your teachings in the field of healing arts helped me to embrace fearless, bold and with resilience the holistic segment, living healing art purposefully, thanks for share your insights with an open mind and heart, mastering the Chinese medicine

methods, Professor thank you for sharing (chi) possibilities in my life.

My special thank you for Dr. Larzelere the methods of acupuncture balance the yin and yang with lightness and mindfulness, your holistic approach is absolutely unique.
The naturopath Krystine kuecha you showed me holistic medicine and the embracing of nature making a positive difference in people's lives, your beautiful female support made the spa business experience possible, you encouraged beautifully, Thank you sister of light for introduce healing herbs, you're a gifted healer, pure essence.

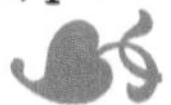

My appreciation M.s Martha and Lilian teller, peer group of elevation, the practice of healing, alignment of chakras and natural healing, I am thankful for all the change that you two ladies brought to my personal life, I am thankful for this light experience.

Mr. Horowitz your contribution to the world of science, supporting communities changing people's life positively, true story, your expertise thought me continue embrace the field of research, above all to do good for others with a positive attitude, you're a real level of effectiveness. Thank you Professor Linstroth your knowledge creates a positive world surround with different cultures, anthropology, greatness, thank you for share the amazon rain forest world and many of your research contributed directly for the natives on the Amazon.

Ms. Dominique Magnon you're gift to the world, your light and your support showed me friendship kindness and true beauty. Thank you.
Ms. Jeanne Hunter you thought me the law of reciprocity, thank you for your teachings and grace.
Mr. Paul Assimacopos I am grateful for the New York community library, writing lessons that motivate foreigners to embrace their passions guiding the literacy, you're a real American greek, Thank you. Efharisto.

Lana Vinhas you're a powerful healer, the alternative healing world brought us together for such unique work to support healing research with love and light always helping people and guide them to the healthy and holistic lifestyle, respect nature and celebrate the vibrational field of life.
To all my patients Thank you for believe in my work and give me the credibility to support during the process of rehabilitation.

A special dedication for all my dear peregrine's friends,
enlightened family through tick and thin beyond this
dimension, the peregrine is never a loner, you never know
what you can manifest until you find the way, my sincere
pray for all of you to find and pursuit your purpose, embrace
the healing journey and continue enlightening and share
blissfulness with the world and nature.
My sincere wishes that you continue find many ways, always
in synchronicity with the stars, and I hope this book guide
you precisely "om" the way.

Preface

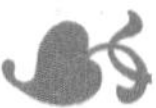

To peruse the field of Alternative medicine and breakthrough
the skepticism of natural healing yet find the roots of
preventive health and continue advocate this art for the
modern generation, the immense benefit of natural
medicine, support the holistic community and embrace the
new development in the segment of alternative medicine,
contribute towards new theories, applying natural healing
methods of alternative healing.
As the advance technology reached the landmark of
modernity influencing with AI, the contribution of natural
healing continue guide healthy communities, supporting
method of natural holistic medicine focused on future
generations with holism methods, preventive medicine and
natural methods that works effectively supporting the
harmonious contact between the individual and nature with
their culture, beliefs and genetics.
I've visited different countries to understand the quality of
life, people's lifestyle, beliefs and their environment.
The modern world experience disconnection with time,
space and human evolution, many are living the intensity of
technology, living the moment is a common expression, the
individual find answers and consistently are living the
oblivious unconscious reactions, emotions, psychology and
physiology, for this sake this book guide readers balance the
state of mind, body and soul with natural healing.

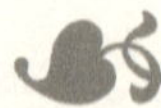

During this research I had the privilege of meeting amazing people of different cultures, beliefs and lifestyle and listen their stories, people are amazing on their own way and this holistic field research became possible because of cultural differences, indeed contributed explore ways of healing, throughout history the holistic conscious lifestyle is a regular practice that allows nature vitally integrates and during this experience I found myself living the holistic life, healing, modify my nutrition, become conscious about my Amazonian life and embrace the minimalistic lifestyle.
For me the hardest part of this research has been living the traveler lifestyle struggling throughout the process breakthrough " my own bubble" and my limited beliefs as well change old pattern, hands on realism and human nature. The overall holistic medicine thought me that people relies on their unique ways to embrace healing and their relationship with nature is crucial, many breakthrough and insights happened during this research, everywhere the world have the unique habitat that support the many way of healing throughout generations these methods of holistic healing innovates as families and communities reach the tree of life with quality of life and methods of survival, explored journey and adventure allows many ways that fully recreate, replace and cope the modern lifestyle with healthier approaches. The alternative medicine is a gift for young generation and the acceptance of natural healing regardless of western or eastern medicine philosophies many doctors and patients everyday embrace the relationship with nature, protecting the natural habitat as well practicing holistic medicine approaching a healthier nutrition, detoxifying the body as well practice mindfulness thriving on nature a better lifestyle.

The adaptation of healthier habits comes from consistency and positive methods, the modification of old patterns, introducing the communication and expression where the elements of nature strengths the body, reverse unhealthy conditions within body and restore the mindset towards a soulfully and mindfully living experience.

The relevance of alternative medicine throughout this time is crucial, apply healthy scientific methods become popular in urban and rural areas to find benefits that develop and better communities, some eco friendly and many primitive concept are adapted as holistic healthy standards sustainably designed as prioritize the holistic preventive healing world, supporting infants and elderlies healthier generations.

To create a world conscious more need to be done and it encouraged me continue the research within theoretical holistic field of holistic preventive healing, many challenges the world experiences on the false illusion of developmental technology, more people are using unhealthy approach, it's time to embrace a healthier life, you can begin this journey today, as well experience a healthier happy life with natural preventive approach of mind and body experience healthier living experience.

The methods encourage people's beliefs bound with nature elevating the mind as well strengths the immunity system combining new ways that prioritize the overall health.

The connection with nature and the methods of mind elevates individual vitality between the scientific pseudo-psychology and physiology, the believes strengths the vital energy within body prioritizing healing and the communication with nature.

The obliviousness response, somatic pain within body conducts the individual sedentary or healthy choices towards a greater understand of their body and the relationship with the emotions and homo sapiens nature.

In conclusion unhealthy people have less interaction with nature, including their eating habits, lifestyle, food supply, cosmetic products and their habits are unconsciously weakening their immune system, the modern male and female find many ways to explore the unnatural appearance as well unhealthy coping and disconnect with nature, mechanism such unrealistic ways elevating the materialistic lifestyle as one way towards overcome somatic pain, the coping mechanism this DNA and age reduce people's vitality comparable with previous generations, people are living the moment of the overwhelmed age of information, yet this can be the healthiest generation when truth people embrace nature. This is the remedy to improve humankind the connection with nature, readapt and recreate with alternative medicine methods towards a healthier life.

The contact with nature influence many towards evolution ways as well connect with significant habitat and preventive healing, releasing the importance of the evolved generation with methods to rectify the emotions and rationalize their communication towards recreate a better experience as the individual as the element of nature reach clarity, integrates and creates healthier experiences.

The science of nature and holistic way of living through the modern world supports longevity, boost body's energy, elevate a healthier mindset and spirit as the need to share and discuss about vitality and healing process aiming a healthier world and generations.

The alternative medicine elevates the communication between the individual and their habitat and reach the purposefully the transparency as well quality of life, communication, introduce different ways of healthy living and reach the identification of a balanced life.

Summary

This book easily guide and motivate the seekers to find ways to communicate with nature and most importantly, achieve inner cure with affirmatives that create a healthy lifestyle. The comprehensive language offers concisely the alternative medicine methodology encouraging the individual develop healing approach ways and conduct their genetic code in relation and connection with nature.

The healing path addresses spirituality and the belief of the individual as well scientifically support the bound that strength with nature many ways to define the dynamic that motivates the individual step up towards self healing, positive experience precisely in the path towards self improvement. This introduction of alternative medicine present methods that breakthrough old patters and somatic pain, heals emotions, refine towards vitality and connect deeply with inner self, let the nature of individual and DNA be the cure as the individual belief well prevent naturally the healthy living of a conscious mind and body.

The book allows the embrace on the recovery road and explore ways of breakthrough and understand old patters coping mechanism with healthy, inspiring and creative ways towards the consistent alternative natural healing practices, revealing the encounter with gravity and the effect of gravity between the cycles of life, exploring the depth of the element of nature and the benefits of nature to the body and mind throughout the experience biofeedback, organic nutrition and finding significant approach towards combine the right minerals and vitamins to balance body's ph and find essential health.

The practice of alternative healing methods will lead to the right frequency where the individual connect with the habitat, the matching frequency between concrete and abstract positive and negative, upwards and downward ratio frequency within universe and its dualities frame to reach the resonance towards the evolved and improved healthy lifestyle, elevating the mind and body, knowing the process and respect the time it will help realizing that now is the moment to balanced and match the frequency.
The relationship with self when focused with the healthier habits improve the individual universe, through affirmation and ability to be proactive, the share of consciousness elevates healthier way to guide the body and mind successfully.
The nature of mind and soul genetically allows the individual receive and perceive nature differently, thriving and achieve happiness in different ways, this guide will give you key that will help you to consciously unlock and release somatic pain with the introduction, the holistic healing will release positively opening a constructive experience as the individual step into the process that will allows them rejuvenate elevate towards a healthier frequency elevating the functionality with natural methods of healing connecting effectively with methods of self improvement allowing the individual feels and consciously choose a healthier life.
The healing simplify the road of recovery, giving the individual closure and completeness helping the embrace bounding with wellness and create a grounded self love and identify the wholistic balance of body, mind and soul.

Table of contents

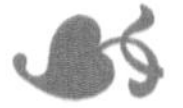

Unveiled The Pure Healing

Alternative medicine guide to share on the way!

RUSIANE ALMEIDA

Chapter 01

The healing Path

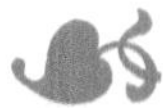

To overcome health issues the solution of the modern world is alternative medicine coping methods with nature, practicing the natural healing medicine positively release body, mind and soul with non invasive methods increase healing and rehabilitation. What Western and Eastern medicine have in common? Both medicine peruse one subject "Treatments" two different ways to approach health yet with accurate science of "Healing and Rehabilitation."

The alternative medicine research facts, diagnosis and causes, involving innovative ways to create new treatment, revealing a greater importance for the individual to embrace preventive medicine. The Alternative medicine is not the woo-woo but a precise science with methods that guide the individual for century towards good health, quality of life and better relationship with nature, it brings values to the sustainable natural environment and the healing consciousness of nature. Its essential for the modern individual to find alternative ways of living towards healthier lifestyle, extend lifespan experience the identity with nature.

The wholistic technology creates healthy methods that overcome diseases through the connection with nature, find benefits about disconnect the individual of the virtual world and brings fully present mind, body and soul with the environment for a better health, reduce sedentary living and increase moments of consciousness towards a healthier generation, approaching the vitality, longevity and living lifestyle of preventive health.

The modern medical field advance with segregate groups investing time and medical researches as advance and innovate treatments, Working through authentic or placebo effects applying methods

that better work for the individual through their identification process with nature, letting nature be thy medicine.
 The truth medicine heals body and mind, support through the recovery and belief ways as the individual and the connection with nature find the best practice that strengthen the immune system, physiology and psychology, the overall wholistic energy field of the individual.
The modern world of stress, virtual technology and unhealthy coping caused millions of people to experience unbalanced lifestyle.
The ability to create healthier path remains with these truth facts, introduce healthier alternative choices, become steady, effective and consistent with the alternative healthy ways, the structure to balance and reverse unhealthy patterns remain in the individual codification of the body, mind and soul.
The alternative medicine viability support different branches of medicine, organically nourishes the vitality of body and mind, it is the way to perceive a healthier body with a positive mindset.
The goal is adapt practical methods to measure health accordingly with the individual RNA, cells and DNA balancing the psychology and physiology adapting a wholistic way " the healthy conscious living" find ways that identify the individual through understand overall uniqueness of hereditary, eating habits and routine familiarizes healthier choices as their own methods of preventive and rehabilitate as the holistic dynamics further surface as the individual explore the overall body, mind and soul and apply healthier choices "the healing path" release the old habits and introduce new healthier habits life approach, regeneration, positive beliefs, adapt a better nutrition and continue develop ways to experience a healthier lifestyle.
To experience a better relationship with nature it is necessary to create, restart and walk a healing path where the individual find the enjoyment with nature as a result reduce inflammation within body, recreate health and address differently unhealthy habits adapting new ways of healing within path that benefits the body, mind and the spirit of the individual.

The way *

The healing path is a journey of emotions and self identification, times positive, times negative, the result is the synchronicity, as a result the feedback essence becomes the individual's action.
As the relationship with nature reinvigorates, the individual finds balance and the outcome of the emotions creates awareness as the state of mind progress " breakthrough" the old patterns and experience healing successfully as part of the identification. Alternative medicine is the method that assist the individual coping healthier and positively.
From the moment the baby born the vital senses connects with the living environment, the sequences of habits is stablished as breakthrough old habits become necessary to create healthier emotions, if not coping healthier it greater aggravates the patterns such as stress, anxiety and depression increase, factual that such way must occur the intervention that reverse toxic habits brings a quieting balanced focused mind elevating self "identity" and self improvement.
On the way, the importance of meditation helps the individual understand the environment, resets mind and body send positive thoughts to rebuild new cells and practice the detachment with the environment thus increasing healing possibilities, reducing increase the nature as balance the a body chemistry response, the overall experience with emotion becomes the essence of the individual. The external environmental is the creator fact that affect and contributes towards action and reaction , balance and reverse fight and flight leveraging on the behalf of mind and body, during healing process nature adjust the response within body and mind vital pulses, decrease or increase homeostasis as a way to balance the physiological and psychological response, the goal is interfere stress hormone (fight and flight) body and mind exposing alternative medicine methods daily to restore body, mind and soul of the individual.

A supportive method strengthens the body and mind and continue positively creating the identification though the road of rehabilitation, familiarize with self as the most effective approach redirect towards a release somatic pain emotions that unconsciously remain and surface towards a self sabotage unhealthy lifestyle, yet with less attachment with the environment and focused consciously in leverage the process towards healthy connection with nature as part of the "ascension.".

Imagine a toddler during the first steps holding father and mother hands acquiring new abilities to practice ahead the training process, the toddler acquire muscle memory and strength, the immunity anti-corps better senses touching, breathing and tasting, the toddler acquires through the five sense resiliency that will safely during the process fight and flight the toddler learn abilities to reverse stress and create strength where finally he finds gravity reaching the main purpose, the toddler wins the battle, the toddler survive by activate the sensory and impulses and coordinate the body and mind, it finally walk the way and this mindset growth on us daily, the toddler learn the walk, the individual practice daily consciously methods of self interests and between gravity and survival, health is the priority. The alternative healing methods helps walk the steps change raising consciousness, increasing awareness, release gravity field, raising the healthy and fulfilling life, as toddler walking memories, it is actions that embrace life and fully shift towards healthier and appreciative ways into well grounded feelings that switch steps towards a balanced life focused on the healthier way forward, releasing good laugh(serotonin) and develop ways that runs better healthier habits switching positively for a greater lifestyle, practicing steps towards a new healthy version of the body, mind and soul, the way increase the immunity choosing the way to practice new habits and connect with the environment positively, increase happiness and release positive contact with the environment substituting nature as through breathing, nutrition, sleep, walking on the grass barefoot, breath and become one with nature.

The primitive survival Homo sapiens dedicate the energy for hunting food(exercise) eat (nutrition) Sleep (rest) the cavern man vitamins and mineral runs through the physiological response and predators fear hides the believe of find meal next day (pray)

It's the practice of meditation that creates homeostasis within body, hugging friends and trees (touch) leverage and release self stronger five sense, through this process perhaps hearing a song or singing a melody, play the instrument is a way to find out about new abilities of your own, running, jumping, swimming etc. activates the body and mind. The way activates the self it does connect with nature and let nature speak to the individual through the desire of nature and feeling as the ocean breeze, it does not matter where you at or which part of the world embrace nature is the only way to release tension within mind, body and soul. Alternative medicine elevates positive feedback helps to release the nervous system with different mindset, the healthy wellbeing is the healing journey aiming to know where to start and how to begin, it creates the first place of consistency stage .

Let it go distraction, living the practice moment of breathing, adapt the comfort of your home, on the beach, parks or mountains be comfortable with yourself, the balance and strengths body and mind reality as the individual resiliently embrace the road beyond limitation and limits.

The breathing is the most important function of the body helps correct the posture, and reduce stress, the air element plays a major role, reversing anxiety, tension and stress, allowing a positive body's language, breathing creates a confident mindset sending oxygenated blood to the brain, inhaling the wellbeing and exhale tension completely, start create alternative ways to breathing , E.g (Thai chi) the art of Thai Chi and different methods elevate body's consciousness and brings the healthy breathing from the lungs to the brain and different organs as well support the practice endure the focus as strength the core revitalizing the body, it works wellness for introverts and extroverts appreciating the practice benefit and move the chi energy and release the stress(stagnated chi) energy that suppresses the immune system.

The posture during breathing elevates and expand a better alignment with the body, techniques of tapping energy within body is a complementary supporting way that alleviates nervous system activate homeostasis within body brings the feeling of becoming present experiencing and connect with body's nature.

The body compass re-adapt new habits, the practice of breathing correctly practice exercise the largest muscle of the body (The diaphragm) breathe the Solar Plexus(Adrenal Gland) the body mechanics aligns with a correct respiration, practice a correct body posture towards a better aligned posture, open up channels of gratitude, it is with arms wide open that the individual reconnect with the inner self.

There's many alternative ways that can be selected accordingly with the individual differences, these activities balance energy level for any given circumstances and the goal remain re-adapt and develop a better identification, managing the increase or decrease of body's energy, redirect finding compatibility with nature as alternative methods helps familiarize and introducing to the relevant way of unleash the healing potential within body, the first communication (communicate body and mind) the essence self, the breathing methods is the path many cycles towards vitality and vibration of life within body and mind is the communication that define nature and creation resembling divinely though(inhale and exhale)

Practice simple exercise such as standup barefoot as feeling grounded both feet together, identify your direction and take a deep breath, let it go through another deep breath, feeling the alignment each breath bring you to the present as you are comfortably letting it go, repeat it as you wish, breathing with posture is a natural ways of alignment as you feel the body shifting according with find ways towards strength the immune system satisfactorily this become practices that connect wellbeing with self (identity) mindfully the focus of the homeostasis effect elevates the mind towards breathing as open up the meridians channels (the system of the body) towards a healthier present body and mindset.

* DNA, Nature and Prevention *

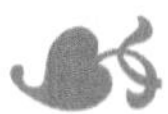

DNA is the unique sequence of life, it defined genetics which predict the individual healing lifestyle experience (genetical code) The print translate generations carrying in and out through the cells the sequence weakening or strengthening the immune system.

The dietary and hereditary plays an important role during (recovery stage) apply alternative methods accordingly with DNA through the elements of nature elements manifest cure and methods of healing. It must be adapted as create the new healthy habits mindset, during healing process crucially recover stages strengthening body, mind and soul. The spirituality of healing is importantly conscious as communicate the language translating body and mind, these beliefs are constructively in adaptation strengthening the DNA code settings and the practices of generations that lead to the individual reconnection with vital energy experiencing the cure of their nature.

The cure of any disease relies within individual gene and the belief on their own capabilities of healing, what can't be cured must be endured, cure will never be present on the incomplete mind, body and spirit.

The alternative medicine is the science that gives the individual methods to complete and reach the wholistic cure of body, mind and spirit.

I was born in the Amazon Rainforest and my identification with natural healing started during Junior High, throughout the biology classes groups explored different interests of spirituality, the living experience in the amazon rainforest is indeed interesting and peculiar, the jungle is wild.

My dear classmate and I created a project where we both
interviewed different healers in our hometown, during the
interviews we find out that their experience and resources was
quite limited, researching their abilities, we dove deeper as we
found ourselves crossing lakes with canoe to interview healers, as
they referred each other based on their own psychic abilities and
communication with nature practices of different beliefs as
alternative methods included varieties of teas, herbal baths,
massages, incense cleanser among plants, during the project we
were introduced to the medicine woman, one of the greatest
native amazonian healer in our hometown, a midwife and native
Amazonian, since the first day we've knocked at her door, and she
answered from her window our project were finally completed, she
managed the healing arts and guided us towards a better
relationship with nature, she thought us about life and spoke the
language of nature, the midwife of our community, a woman of
simplicity, graceful as her warmness attracted many people
searching healing, her daily life were healing, she was very busy,
blessing the children, families, anointing the sick, blessing
mothers and fathers. She allowed nature speak through her body,
mind and soul.
After significant breakthroughs in my personal life, the field of
therapeutics treatments growth deeply on my concept , my
experiences within Amazon with a medicine woman significantly
made realize self improvement healing.
Later I started realize that alternative healing goes beyond, it is
the exact science with methods that manage the cure.
As the introduction of the holistic lifestyle, the healing path
method continued as healing arts that highly improved the
harmony of the one with nature and better understand holistic
medicine, embracing healing and cure the journey created
through new beliefs transforming old beliefs towards self love, self
realization and connection with nature. It does create quality of
life nature is cure regardless of the environment.
The re-adaptation of emotionally, physically, psychologically or
spiritually, reveal the natural principles of preventive medicine
within soul, body and mind, healing will allow the embrace of the
process with a positive mindset, resiliently towards the overall
wellbeing of our modern society

The theoretic studies in preventive medicine of the health segment motivated me continuously explore possibilities to help people access a healthier lifestyle, as a woman in science embracing the modern field of holistic medicine and therapeutic interested in the studies of different cultures as well understand habits and the habitat supporting technologies that lead towards the positive society.

The path have two important facts (the nature and the nature of the individual) the identification of concrete ways of living and abstract ways of living, studies towards the individual and the identification with nature, the contact with nature and the environment and the supports of the survival of mankind, the genes of the individual pure healing and recovery stages within body physiology, biochemistry and psychology. The wellbeing that enable the individual towards thrive in different habitat, includes different space, region and the wellness wellbeing experience, the alternative medicine is the channel that embrace communication (the individual and nature) the connection that increase with the purpose to enhance the immunity and resilience of the individual, it recreate and fight diseases, reverse toxicity within cellular level, aid rehabilitative process and support longevity.

As technology advance and explore different models of sustainable habitat in the world, nature does protect the overall wellbeing of humankind, the belief remains prioritizing each individual DNA, as people identify with the uniqueness of themselves and find health and a better lifestyle to the way that activate longevity through consciousness of (habits and habitat) nature is an integrative extension of body and mind as Alternative medicine is crucial for this communication, mates connects through their healthier belief and magnetism, the nature resets deeply, elevates healthy way to process the mind.

Alternative medicine for patients during rehabilitation reveals a continue process towards synchronicity with body, time, consistence, mind and resting.

The rehabilitation process begins with tracking daily improvement mapping continuously the cycle of detoxification.

The consistency during detox (decluttering) rest (sleep Reset) when followed these simple daily reinforcement healthy steps aid the process, tree important facts that supports basic body mechanics such as the human ability to deal with gravity and daily actions. The injury affects body overall wellbeing therefore before the injury occurs the body mechanics and the habitat of the individual predicts endless probabilities (the body awareness) eminent with the environment, during sport events the athlete training memorized actions (body mechanics) the central nervous system it's is aware of the body and the environment therefore during a somatic stress, perhaps exhaustion ,time management and consistency (the performance) and poor sleep hours(body reset) body reflex the impact and trauma experienced on the range of motion, the athlete restricts and affect the body awareness causing the injury from the physical to the unconscious mind, it's within DNA that the nature of the individual aware the resiliency of the body.

The athlete is a great example of conscious body and mind prevention(the awareness) it's from a great odds that the individual experience an injury in daily basis routine or at work, we are all susceptible, it makes each of us the athlete of our own daily journey, as dealing with regular fight and flight and freeze responses. All the system of the body have important command from the central nervous system and prevention, it lead through a healing process of positive feedback, the homeostasis within body follow the DNA message as the synchronicity of the overall system of the body, vital pulse and stabilization.

The effect of alternative healing elevates the resilience and better communicate between the individual nature and the habitat (nature) by integrate the communication between the physical and the mind to maintain the balance .

The wholistic overview and the overall wellbeing of the individual from one road and system to achieve healing, identify the habitat as a natural way, reconnect and readapt sending positive neurotransmitters strengthening the mindset and regenerate.

* Spirituality is the cure*

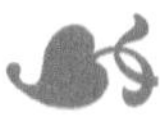

The path of happiness relies on the healthy body, mind and soul, the balance and synchronicity of the individual's nature is the natural state of manifestation.
The spiritual belief of the individual is the foundation, the basics of the primary connection of the individual and the path of spirituality (mindfulness) theses beliefs of life are stablished from a state of blissfulness or fear, the connection with deep emotion and reasoning of the human nature creates spirituality.
All religions are good, religion is the mankind supportive ways towards vitality and the belief through (life and death)
The spirituality support the individual release of resentment, blockages of chi(vital energy) and through the spiral of emotions, as the nature of the individual finds balance spirituality the core and guidance, towards manifestation of healthy lifestyle, wellbeing and quality of life.
The synchronicity of feelings and rationality connects to beliefs positively, the alternative healing is the science of transformation that evolved from the overall wholistic towards wellbeing and the art that enhance body's vitality.
The natural medicine is the remedy that connect the high performance of body and mind, the holistic process activate the essence of the individual. (Soul) , enhancing the immunity as well strengthens the individual immune system reliance, retaining information within body resiliently, increasing physiology, including the hormonal changes, elevating psychology and physiology, regenerating the human capabilities to achieve a healthier life.

The modern technology continues exploring new ways to influence the human body, mind and soul.

It's important that the individual experience the environment and increase consciousness for a better habits and recreate the habitat. The daily practice of spirituality is a way to appreciate the law of nature and the spiritual belief of the cure for any diseases, the natural alternative preventive methods is humankind path towards evolution and the elevation of a healthy way of living. The increase of alternative methods is the solution to reverse diseases, unhealthy habits and influence body's physiology and psychology positively towards a pure natural conscious living, the practice with nature spirituality heals the body and cure the mind, nature elevates necessary beliefs on the individual to heal body and mind and encourage towards a balanced law of self improvement , nature and the universe.

The habitat of the individual changes accordingly with the consciousness of the individual, the spiritual consciousness cure old habits and old beliefs, this self awareness leads towards a well balanced journey where motivation, inspiration and affirmation begins to create a better healthy path re-directing as an effective compass of self healing.

The body and mind guides naturally towards the individual spiritual beliefs, if the body experience weakening within immune system, alternative medicine inspire the individual to continue practices daily to enhance the immune system increasing consciousness of body and mind.

To modify the individual habits and habitat it's important the awareness and understanding that each singular have its own change and healing process, as a result the practice of become conscious of old habits become crucial.

The resilience is the key that associate beliefs of a healthy way of living, identify the natural genetic that connect and easily support a better way of quality of life, acceptance and reflect wholistic within body and mind.

* Decluttering the thought*

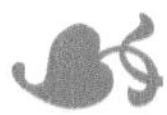

How many times consciously you check and review your inner compass?

The inner compass is the time of the individual and during healing this process adapt nature through walking the path of a positive lifestyle, it is necessary to eliminate toxic habits, detoxify and clear the energy absorbing through life (decluttering) the life energy of the individual from the essence and the five senses, at cases that elevate the essence and the crucial decluttering process with the the guide compass, it help create and review body's wellbeing such as taste, smell, hearing, sight and touch. Ask yourself these simple such questions... What am I seeing recently?

Does my sight elevate myself? What am I eating? Does that taste fresh and nourish my body? Does my environment smell fresh as nature? Am I listening beautiful songs oftentimes and reinforcing positive affirmation? and the final question Am I present in my universe?

These questions helps the individual find the inner compass and understand its own surrounds.

By review nature five senses habitually, this practice amplify and encourage self beliefs towards a healthier path, the importance of a healthy compass helps define healthy ability and restore the connection with truth self, the inner compass isn't about your connection with your loved ones, friends, co-workers and socials but the connection with yourself (identity)

I am the creator of my own life, I am a master of my inner compass and I am manifesting healing.

Resetting the body comes from a settle of interaction between (adaptation, re-adaptation and surrender). The decluttering process activates the healthy way of living, restore homeostasis and the restful positive feedback of body and mind reaching deeply the soul, the decluttering helps the individual let it go the egoistic matter and reach the nirvana.

To enhance body's mechanics towards a healthy , healing and reduce inflammation within body as well regulating blood pressure, creates a steady function of heart rates, mindfulness and homeostasis. One must create the letting go decluttering mindset. To be, or not to be, the road leads towards the accountability and breakthrough old habits reaching a healthier life as continue rise above choosing healthier ways to reach clarity through the process of better control and make positive choices of body mind and soul. Learn to set your time and dedicate consistently for the alternative practice that regularly supports your body and mind positively.
It is important the connection with a positive mindset that practice, creative wellbeing ways and energize the vitality of the body and mind. The time of appreciate the inner self for greatest nature, the moment you decide to walk a new path, living pure healing and leaving behind the unconscious restrictions, practice consciously becoming present, making time to find positive choices and new passions as fully embrace life.
The practice of decluttering adjust and stabilize the positive scale, focusing and let go distraction as resonate clarity of mind (thoughts) and proactive healthier body.
The practice of healthier habits starts fully dealing with emotions effectively, the understanding of the emotion condition better triggers, reprogram better choices that overcome and annulling previously one, identify how these decisions are supporting yourself make better choices and introduce dosage of self awareness,(self-love) the transformation towards healthier habits. On the road learn to be one with nature feeling the body, stretching and create the particles of life, alternative ways to feel alive with nature supporting the process of recovery, and continue raising level (leverage) certainty within body, finding healing benefits the process the growth consciousness and manifest the healthy and constructive mindset.

The body is made of 80% of water, water shapes within vessel, the ability to be a constructive vessel lies within individual, shaping the emotion and the will of the individual towards better choices (the rationality) exercise the connection and create ways to relate with time, more the individual practice self belief more the individual raise with empathy, consistent ways to continue the self improvement practice as positively shift towards healing and self discovery.

Through nature it improve new beliefs, declutter old thoughts, when applied consistently toxic cycles are released throughly better ways of living, it does require the adaptation of self discipline, the well defined ways to manifest healing.

To understand, release and reconnect first adapt better habits (the awakening) Appreciate the frequency(starting point) the present rising and elevating respect between self, nature and universe (self reflection) towards healthier decisions and choosing the way of living, improving therefore the lifestyle and adapt to the greater frequency through nature. It activate the higher frequency within body, manifesting fulfillment (kundalini) alternative healing is a practiced when applied habitually strength mind, body and soul. The alternative medicine results into restore and growth, the evolution of nature within individual vassal, exercising the chi force (Body's vitality) as the remedy of evolution among other practices yoga, breathing, mantra, energy frequency, acupuncture, massage therapy, osteopathy, chiropractic, homeopathy, naturopathy, Thai chi, nutrition, nature grounding, sun bathing, baths, stones, nutrition, pray and practice of your own beliefs etc...The positive mindset restores the overall frequency of body, mind and soul (wholistic methods).

Decluttering old thoughts habitually leads towards a healthy experience and elevate significantly the pure essence of the soul, felling healthy and alive.

To start familiarize with decluttering first return to the origin connecting with earth, restoring and select a new habit as the meditative state to manifest cure, create a new frequency through the environment and redirect with nature.

The environment is the middle point as between sunset and sunrise the redirect of the energy attract closer the nature, strengths five senses and open the healing channels concept (the road of recovery).

On the road you find the uniqueness of each individual and its purpose that embrace the moment and develop empathy, adapt effective ways towards the constructive mindset as well releasing and revealing emotions. The nonsenses of old beliefs adapting a positive mindset bringing to the surface the power of transformation, living meaningfully, substantially as well accomplishing a mindful shifting from the negative to the positive perspective of body, mind and soul.

As the healing practice progresses, prepare strategically ways to reset and create self respectfully, identifying the laws of healing present within body, nature and the universe.

The healthy healing road reinforce to beware of the environment, be present and overcome the path positively.

The energetic field is a reminder to the individual to always surround yourself with healthier experience, choose your healing therapist wisely and identify the presence of healing growth beyond of any given circumstance, healing is important and the moment of shift happens when a new level progresses towards a positive and better experience.

Chart of healthy habit:
 Practice healthier habits tracing your chart, review old habits using this chart to accomplish a healthier lifestyle such as (Quit smoking, weight loss, reverse stress etc...)
review the graphics weekly and periodically
In the scale of 1 to 10 check the improvement of your overall lifestyle.
1Nutrition 1 2 3 4 5 6 7 8 9 10
2 Workout 1 2 3 4 5 6 7 8 9 10
3 Mindfulness Meditation 1 2 3 4 5 6 7 8 9 10
4 Connection with nature 1 2 3 4 5 6 7 8 9 10
5 Healthy choice (________________) 1 2 3 4 5 6 7 8 9 10
6 Relationships 1 2 3 4 5 6 7 8 9 10
7 Work satisfaction 1 2 3 4 5 6 7 8 9 10
8 Stress relief 1 2 3 4 5 6 7 8 9 10
9 Sharing positively 1 2 3 4 5 6 7 8 9 10
10 Motivation 1 2 3 4 5 6 7 8 9 10

A) Rate your lifestyle with an accurate number
B) Practice a new belief e.g (Do not check 10 if you find yourself eating compulsively nutrition checks neither check 2 if you workout 5 times on the week and believe that isn't enough)
C) The chart balance the cycle you can continue shift these number orders as you prioritize
D) Reward yourself during the process with 1/2 point on the scale. adjust, elevate and decrease towards number "8" alignment.

0________________5____________8__________ 10 9I 8I 7I 6I 5I 4I 3I 2I

   Your goal is reach 8 on the scale
   1/2 point are given for the weekly consistency
    1 point mean one number shifted in the healthy scale.

Chapter 02

Down the road

Life down the road happens meaningfully as the individual surrender and recognize the moment of self improvement and create new possibilities to manifest healthier emotions and freedom.

To learn the magical journey of transformation self love is practiced in order to release old patterns and resentments, as the individual becomes aware of their emotion, cooping healthier as a way to familiarize the inner self and approach the road of a healthier and well guided body, mind and soul. It does consciously reach positive structure, grounding healthier with nature.

The therapeutic treatments review improvements in different session and analyze the positive feedback restoring health as the message within body and mind change creating homeostasis and balancing physiology and psychologically on the road of recovery, the releasing toxic patterns and negative emotions towards a constructive mindset establish a successful and healthier lifestyle.

The healing process is a positive feedback that restores and resets body, mind and soul, assuring and activate the overall frame of a well balanced energy healing.

The alternative medicine is the way forward down the road of recovery and work effectively towards improve and coping healthier body, mind and soul.

* The individual road*

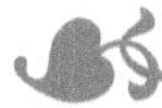

The spiritual, emotional and mental is the main codes of each individual (the identity), the experience registered and recorded is the profile necessary for the body, mind and soul, its an upgrade that reach the wellbeing stage, the wholistic approach that helps to reach the restoring stage of the the energetic field of balance. When an injure occur within body, mind or soul the brain blocks, numbs and rejects pain going to the (obliviousness) this healing process takes places as body resets the emotions and create the overall experience healing consciously therefore the unconscious mindset sleeps within cellular level (body).
We haven't been designed to overcome injury and pain and for this process to happen the individual must be conscious of the oblivious, the evolution readapts naturally as attach the individual on the gravitational field, the daily routine of abstract and concrete navigates towards conscious and unconscious that create muscles memories and resiliency in different ways.
The action and reaction is the sequence of the alternative medicine and unlock the obliviousness of the mind healing process, this awareness of the injury stage when happen the individual down the road becomes familiar with the truth self and stop resistance of the healing process, release cause and effect of the emotion, progressing the mindset freely towards a healthier habit (redemption) when the body exhausts physically and spiritually resembles, the goal of restoration of the vital energy and transcend the emotion, spirituality and the inner nature.
 The healing path is one of the most transformational and uplifting path that creates new possibilities towards a healthier life.
The healing leads to the existence of healthier spirit, mind and body.

* **Down the road and gravity***

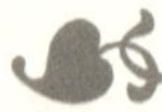

The surrender process helps to embrace down the road of the recovery, the wholistic awareness reconnect each individual towards a healthier and greater experience balancing towards wellbeing .
The meaning of living a healthier life relies on the balanced emotion and rationality, the remedy is the adapt of the genuine mindset and understand the effect of gravity.
The growth is a inevitable process e.g (seeds transcend plants and the growth on the surface of earth as the result) down the road, ascending body, mind and soul is the body essence designed uniquely to recreate growth.
The vibration of the atmosphere and the nature phenomena is the force of energy that elevates the field accordingly with the energy of the individual.
The healing happens when the individual overcome the habitat attachments, gravitating consciously positively transforming old habits, healing the body and create new experience towards a healthier lifestyle.
The natural field of energy breakthrough the gravitational energy, the inner vitality and the capability that body, mind and soul naturally creates to reverse self sabotage presented in the environment.
To adapt body, mind and soul towards a healthier lifestyle and create awareness practice connection with nature as the vital process of life, exercise steady movement completing with self, embrace the divine force and law of nature, growing, healing and regenerate through the process respecting the nature's cycle.

The body (the vessel) and the absorption of the environment, its important to recreate positive feedback, regenerate and nourish (healing process) elevating the immunity as combine cleansing, detox, clean water, herbs and plant base to create a physical balance.

The energetic healing is the process where nature phytochemical and photosynthesis creates a positive feedback rising biochemistry level within body, mind and soul.

The gravitational field and its elements compress and expand in the matter, down the road accumulating emotions, injuries, somatic pain and regrets manifest as aging process in the body, mind and soul, alternative healing release stagnated chi, glands blockage (chakras) and breakthrough gravity(time and space) elevating the healthier perspective of body, mind and soul growing and shaping towards release the emotion.

The body consciously or unconsciously at time at least once will experience an injury, the injury comes from 50% the effect of emotion or 50% from the cause, these habits developed throughout time within habitat communicates with the environment, the stagnation happens when the body and mind refuse to heal properly opposing to recognize the natural law of nature (action and reaction.) The healing can become a long road if there's no intention, action and manifestation, healing can be an illusory description if there's no consistency on the practice (action) the healing path is a natural growth.

The road is the life path that creates vitality within body elevating the intention through nature's cycle, embracing the natural process of life and the alternative medicine.

Each individual carries within the DNA the inner compass of healing that leads them towards self improvement, healing , growth, releasing, shifting and lead towards a better healthier life. Alternative healing supports the transformational experience, helps eliminates pain shifting to the appreciation of the process and find the belief of the individual, gaining clarity towards a healthier positive rising.

Walking the path brings consciousness of the gravitational field as the present action and reaction, breakthrough past resentments and information that holds body, mind and soul.

The gravity blocks the matter creating magnetic attachments, the goal of alternative healing is breakthrough vicious cycle, guiding the individual gently towards a positive life with the alignment of the body, mind and the soul.

The teachings of Hippocrates challenges the individual to fully embrace nature, the human development comes from nature and is founded in nature, alternative medicine strengths the healthy cycle resiliently healing the cause or the emotional effect.

The positive mindset creates a survival mode that motivates the individual towards self Improvement, the positive mindset releases habits from the mind, certainly working on unchanged mindset, reversing and embracing the earning of be healthy, releasing distractions and introduce the control of old habits, learning the significance of positive, inspirational process, find healing, practice of self love and explore new ways of living a healthy lifestyle, (the elevation of the soul.)

"The only thing that is ultimately real about your journey is the step that you taking at this moment that's all there ever is real"
Eckhart Tolle

Be comfortable with yourself, embrace the ability to walk down the road with a present mind accepting , respecting with self love and self worth.

The road of self improvement comes from mind, body and soul resulting from the soul print.

The moment that the individual nature embrace the greater five sense perception touching, breathing,listening, tasting,seeing and feeling becomes a total reality, the journey manifesting the livelihood essence.

The practice of healing art, release stress and improve the vitality tuning the emotions laugh, breathing and exercise, the body and mind knows what works breaking old habits, we are programmed to evolve, constantly.

How does the mind reacts?

 According with the theory of the mind, the individual grasp a rational reality with the basic questions What is this? Or what is happening? It is the nature of the individual question and accept a former concept with an easier explanation as become is the belief or the way of living life, the belief relies on the comfortable answer (self creation) the healing process regenerates mind, body and soul.

To receive the environment as the communicator, the scenario of learning rise on the magnetism through a greater level in the development of self healing , the habitat project the overall state of body, mind and soul. The nature is the dosage needed to walk the concept openness, steady and dedication.

The acceptance of gravity reduces the frustration, as nature reverse feelings, many are living victim of the gravitational field and unconsciously self sabotage the environment, challenging gravity, therefore the gravity is the grounding point of mankind, when the single element accept the creator essence disease are reversed within body through methods of health transformation, decoding DNA code as healthy and cured individual.

The road of ethical, moral and heavenly correct is the journey composed of beliefs, the beliefs are the roots of the cause and the effect, reflecting personal records of life such as feelings and experiences within body and mind, what the individual believe becomes the truth, elevates the emotion and believe in self development as the thriving experience.

The alternative healing supports the practice of positive belief eliminating obstacles down the road, on the mind towards and elevating life .

The process of change requires a dynamic, practice, familiarization as the change of season in such meaningful experience, walking the road reveal a greater understand of self (self awareness) down the road you will get familiar with nature, and nature vibrates inside and outside on the five senses creating positive emotions . There's always an alternative way to make life healthier.

Take a deep breath inn, imagine yourself walking on the perfect
scenario, on the beach feeling the sand, experience the grass,
anywhere and everywhere that best works for you, now feels
barefoot, grounding earth and effectively you can find yourself
thriving with nature with an open heart and beautiful smile, living
the present moment .
The communication developed during healing must be focused on
affirmation, innovation, supporting and guidance towards
resilience, healing is the belief, intention and manifestation, pray
completes the belief system of the individual (find your healing
language) , let nature be the medicine and the body and mind
maintain this communication with nature throughly directly and
indirectly. The healing must be constant as the notes played
towards self improvement, the language and the note that better
resonates during synchronicity, the healing sound it's within you,
let the eco of the consciousness of the universe wave the vibration
of the present moment within universe, the individual's alternative
methods endure on the genes and support the message
differently, it's on the way, every individual uniqueness speak
meaningfully carrying abilities, goals and purpose towards the
genetic code of meaningful life.
The method of decluttering starts with creative space and embrace
new way ahead, the assertive way to make healthier decision, find
new choices and walk the duality paths (right or wrong) rising on
the surface challenging gravity, accepting and readapt through a
greater and significant way forward, rising on the path is the way
forward breaking patterns shaping towards living heaven on the
earth (nirvana) releasing the vibration is the better version of you,
living the gifted life is the essence as walk the healing road is the
practice of vitality and connect with balance and clarity, it become
truthful with the self and manifest the reality(the soul awareness)
living with respect and certainty. A modern pavemented road is
the easy road, the modern world offers endless possibilities, to be
creative, inspirational and growth let your body raise such as lotus
flowers, dahlias, plumeria, peony, orchids and roses like flowers
nourish yourself meaningfully with the vital healing, let the
universe rise from within manifesting light rising morning
melody, birds recognize the habitat, observe, listen touch and let
the heart melody sing your journey.

To advocate alternative healing in the modern world requires a method that works for everyone effectively, nature is the only channel that supports a sincere and positive communication as healing comes from the restoration of the soul.

The reality of body, mind and soul is the constant change of evolutionary process through space and time channeling the universe and the individual (the force of spirituality)

There's alternative ways to find clarity and motivate towards a healthy way as growths happens on the unconditional flow, reaching beyond of body naturally accepting the mind capabilities to reach its full potential elevating towards a sincere soul, becoming the awaken as appreciate every morning, conducting effectively the ride, imagine living joyfully with a grateful heart managing the emotion successfully.

As you find out more about the way, observe steps that track the pavemented road (modern world) adding new process that calculates positively each contrast, images, feelings and experience, healing restore the individual releasing the unnecessary accumulated over time, finding fulfillment, substitute the somatic pain towards a transformational lifestyle, healing childhood, development phases of adulthood.

The individual must heal, reflect the vital pulses release the pain, restore the inner essence, release emotions as the most beneficial alternative practices of healing release the pressure of the gravitational field within body and mind.

To find the essence of alternative practices create a moment where healing becomes a priority towards the elevation.

The goal is to develop a creative road that helps the individual identify with their own essence creating a positive reflex and conduct body, mind and soul healthier.

Let's Improve the focus on the way, achieve new goals, experience healing as well living a fulfilling life.
Select seven colors
1.Purple
2.Blue
3.Green
4.Yellow
5.Orange
6.Pink
7. Red

____

____

____

____

____

____

Write down seven unnecessary thoughts that sabotage your plans and stop your growth, side with goals to be completed meanwhile reversing the self sabotage

____

A) Layout your circle of solution.
B) Divide seven equal parts inside the circle.
C) Place a moving arrow in the middle.
D) Write down seven Your seven goals, filling each space within circle with your goals
E) colors the circle accordingly with the colors of each number.
F) Spin the arrows to start.
G) Concentrate in your goal, let the arrow tells you the one goal to start today.
You can use the wheel every time you need to complete your goal, be effective and focus on a positive healthier mindset.

____

____

____

____

____

____

 Now on the same dynamic let's find the alternative medicine
practice that works best for you.

Select seven alternative practice that you wish to experience in the
next tree months.

Choose one color for each practice
 E.g.(Yoga-Detox- Thaichi- acupuncture- massage - Ayurveda -
chiropractic adjustment - osteopath - sauna etc...)

Write it down seven healing practice to experience physically,
emotionally and spiritually fulfillment.

Select and match colors within circle, spin the arrow and practice
daily until healing been accessed.
Work weekly and observe the results.
Recreate as many times as you please.
 Life is happening for you now.

Chapter 3

Fresh Lemonade for body mind and soul

"When life give you lemons, make yourself the best lemonade"
Begin fresh, start in the morning with a relaxing and detoxifying
body and mind, take a minute to listen the universe, the vibration
towards a healthier mind, vibrate the essence and vitality, plays
the note of synchronicity with the universe appreciating all living
being frequency. The natural properties present in nature supports
and strength the immune system, antioxidants and phytochemical
and the biochemical compound supports the connection with
nature and enhance the creativity towards creation. The way of
consciousness regenerate body's energy is amplifying the
frequency, the density energetic field of body, mind and soul
beginning the insightful state, meditative mindset and positive
frame of mind. Practice nature and nourish the essence. As a
mother during pregnancy and overcoming the hormonal changes,
the experience blossoming and growth, as the concept of
experience the change and embracing the body, creating a
healthier approach and motivate thyself to start with small dosage,
as a weight loss positive change and significantly reaching the
healthier frame consistently, detoxing and practicing love as the
creative ways to be fulfillment with motherhood, experiencing
body and mind as nurturing the spirit. The struggled of my
pregnancy changed my life positively and the effect growth
sincerely on myself where I found dedicating to the field of
Alternative medicine, eventually became the sincere expression of
change, the best lemonade, fresh towards new habits, motivating
positive habits and habitat that inspired as well influenced the
connection, positive emotion and the environment, (frame of
vibration)

* **The Elements** *

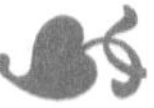

The connection with the matter is presented within the elements; electrons, neutron, cations and protons adding and subtract the atom. The biochemistry define physical energy, understand the element shifts the perspective conditioning the nature within body e.g (switch eating habits for a healthier habits requires add and subtract chemical compound according with the mineral and vitamins) the gene continue thrives in group, humanity thrive towards anything that inspire and connect them individually with the element of nature through the calculation standards of group and habitat.

The element in synchronicity connects the body and mind on the existence (psychology and physiology) with the nature divisions and duality eg: male and female hormones is the synchronicity that procreates life.

The elements shifts within body manifesting the emotional positive balance (serotonin) or stress (cortisone) habits are the repetitive cycle of the chemical compound within body, the alternative way to balance the chemistry adding the element of nature thus the elements is crucial to release inflammation within body, throughout ph process scale (acidity and alkaline), the importance of alternative healing through balance the PH within body. The elements of nutrition merge the meridians and channel the circulating body's synapse with the chemical compounds.

 The electrolytes, antioxidants such as lemons, berries and greens aid the process readapt a way to rejuvenate the body cells.

The holistic medicine stimulates the nature elements within body, shifting the PH manifesting as an energetic restructure of organic compound of vitality, what you feed your body with conscious decision that you make towards a detoxifying and cleansing experience strength the individual genetic structure.

The body's meridian is vital, reset of the meridians and the communication with the organs manifest body's vitality and the pulse of the universe within body, mind and soul.

Practicing detoxifying within cellular level, rejuvenates the structure when life gives you lemons learn how to process the shift action and reaction of the universe within life reality.

* **Pure Hydrogen** *

To prepare a lemonade is required a special compound the difference between citrus and sugar.
The natural sugar compound of honey neutralize the citrus, preparing a lemonade also requires a temperature, during the process feels the vibration, the refreshment of organic ingredients, select the jar and start cut the lemons in half, divide them and squeeze. Feel the squeeze quality of the lemon juice, process in magnitude, the citrus of tree lemons can half the jar as pouring the water, alternating the structure, add your favorite taste and add ice.
The lemonade is a great examples of alternate the PH, change the essence and balance the dosage as feeling the molecule structure. A dosage of love never fails, appreciation increase water molecule structure, sugar and lemons contribute to a healthier alkaline fresh healing body's PH
 To create a fresh lemonade add lemons, fresh water ph and natural sweetener (honey, agave, cane) cleanse the body naturally with nature, option the organic, freshly flavored season and combine the freshness of the lemon preparing the lemonade serving fresh for any occasion, refreshment for body and mind, recognize the freshness within chemical compound elevating the energy and boosting the mood as well finding new ways to experience a fresh lemonade during detoxification.

The Pure Healing detoxification PH*

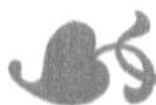

The appreciative art of the sour taste, the lemon juice concentrates acidity within PH that reverse chemistry within body activating healing process.

The alternative therapeutics supports the healing shift, the core essence of the natural chemical compound aids the body balancing the PH, the goal is support the alkaline ph scale crossing the acidity phase within body, release toxins ,healing within PH level transforming the guts (second brain) as well the first brain healing synapse. The overall deeply body, mind and soul transcending towards a balanced pure healing.

The natural process works to reach the upward shift within body, mind and soul translating the DNA code properly with the frequency of nature and the physiology of the individual.

The regression within body slows down the natural cellular level, detoxify release the inflammation, creates new cells, multiply and adjust as cleansing body toxins, elevating the frequency elevates healthier cells, the release of somatic pain frequency within body creates within cellular level wellbeing, body's PH balances energy.

 The most important phase of the healing process through holistic medicine approach and stimulate the cells, balance the outside elements, shifting in single dosage strengthening the cellular level that makes 80% of water effectively tune the body and mind.

The wholistic process works in integration of biochemistry and physiology.

The mind consciousness during cycles, regenerates the individual evolving through biological life cycle and cells cycle producing a healthier lifestyle

To make a lemonade activate the lemon PH, observe, temperature, chemistry and the relevance of time that may take to the maximize fresh juice, extracts the lemon peels and create the lemonade. The perfect fresh lemonade is well measured on the quantity of lemon and honey, the pollenate flower makes the ideal nourishment to balance PH producing the truth essence of the fresh lemonade, the key to create a full jar of lemonade is not raise the water but keep the consistency of the lemon PH, natural chemistry balance elements, natural fresh juices well balanced reverse acidity within body, it can range from different sources (pineapple, mint, wheatgrass, kombucha, strawberries, apples, oranges etc...) Varieties of blend makes well balanced PH flavor, alternative ways to accelerate healing and manifest the healthier life, juicing is the cleansing way, through different fruits, vegetables and electrolytes elements are balanced creating the ideal body's physiology measuring water approximately 50% to 78% of H_2O within human body including balancing hormone, the process of detox require a better intake of water, the significance of water within body to reverse inflammation and transforms the body and restore.

A pure and clean water elevates the PH within individual body, immunity system highly appreciates, a healthy PH thrives communities around the world, H_2O element significantly increase a well balanced lifestyle.

The conservation of water balances the energetic polarities on earth.

 The clean environment leads towards healthy a positive body and mind, water is the healer, tribes around the world crosses continent thriving to the compound of h2o molecule to regenerates cells, the better water filtration, conservation and filtration supporting individuals to thrive the alternative nature. The importance of elements ionizes and transform acidity to the healthier alkaline body's hydrogen refreshing body mind and soul as well inspire a positive lifestyle cycle, making the harmony between the elements of nature and the nature of the individual. The lifestyle builds up longevity as alternative medicine support the overall body, mind through the physicality and abstraction, reversing diseases.

As nature speak the language of life, the cure is present within
nature as the individual body, mind and soul resiliency is
connected within element.
There's many methods of cleansing the uniqueness comes from
value the balance, makes fresh and above of all manifest positive
healing within body.

Chapter 04

Upward Frequency

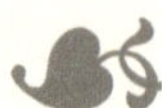

What does make the body vibrate? Movement, the body nature is constantly active and through the resting pulse of gravity and matter is the steady point that frequency of life, the nature silence the echo of existence making particles alive.
The preventive medicine protects the " essence" life's vitality and excitement.
The equation is the movement, time and balance, the dance between life and death, the frequency matches livelihood, emotions and rationality.
What does make life's tick?
Is there a path of frequency that elevates the emotions's cycles, evolve, creates, rebuild as well goes through duality death, destruction, disadvantages all the way towards a virtuous being of frequency. The sound of life is the vibration of the heart pulse and the warmness of human nature, what makes the reality tick as the single element on the earth is the steady lively flow.
What does makes the resonance combines the movement and reach the frequency of attraction?
The consciousness of the being is to be alive!
The code of nature is existence from the Homo sapiens evolution to the human frequency and has been right and wrong decoded to create the better version of self and constructively the " human nature" resonance as the individual free will ticks and uplift life trough the habits and the habitat and continuously plays the constructive source of natural elevation.

The habits is the balance, equalize vibration within individual resonance, it takes frequency to be manifested and balance new habits revitalize a better experience transform destructive nature to productive nature, habits conduct productive as the destructive reach the balance within source of nature vibrating each elements towards life and the ability to communicate the element of nature as well restoring the living particles of the movement as adapting the pulse through a healthier life.

The motion is the frequency between downward and upwards frequency, the unique beat of frequency, relies on the habitual sound, the knowing emotion and the unknowing emotion and body's energy.

The modern technology advanced the field to measure these frequencies on the nature of the individual and the nature, analyzing motions and emotion within body and mind translate the physicality, the frequency of the soul frequency measured through the vitality and the branch of alternative medicine that explore methodology enhancing precise balance of human health, measuring body's energy, screening minerals and vitamins the overall balanced body's pulses assuring regeneration producing body's capabilities to produce and release energy balanced that elevate towards a frequency of life, evolving and pulsing towards a healthier life.

To activate healing the individual must elevate five senses frequency naturally, the individual practice healthy methods that habitually elevates and evaluate restoring the field of energy existent within body. The practice of the principle restore body's energy and evaluate nature ethically on the frequency, the western medicine and eastern medicine researches maintain the core to reset balance within human health.

Human energy is registered within the cellular level, DNA sequence alternate, predicts and modify the energetic field between deep and superficial frequency.

To endure energy its important to understand slow motion, elevation frequency and equalize frequency throughout longevity, the resilience, self preservation, reliance, morals, ethics, sexual instinct and social instinct IQ,EQ, the living being survive on the earth relying in the conscious attraction of the element,

as synchronicity creates meaningful vibrations through the
energetic field, the family procreation through the magnetism
field is the the natural state of upward frequency the individual
nature and nature (instinctual) of two people in harmony.
To evaluate the modern living frequency and the concept of life
throughout the cycle of life extended within the meridian the
elements and frequency as a result creating existence through the
primitive life, evolving, vibrating consciousness, the healing is the
evolution of humanity, the balanced body frequency transcending
between upward and downward frequency well balanced towards
elevate "Thyself"improving the overall body and mind, the goal is
activate healing, elevate the nature of the individual healing,
include the balance of Alter EGO, breakthrough the old for the
better version of the mind and body.
The state of body, mind and soul reality vibrates a pure tone and
this order shift energy the precise math of body pulse, and placed
with individual way to reach the nature as the detachment pulse
helps reach the truth essence of life, when reached with precision
all that remain is divinity of self, healing and nirvana.

* **Elevating Frequency** *

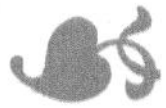

Life from the spiritual point of view, the spiritual practice elevates the frequency of the individual's virtues as betterment of the path, redemption is the pure healing frequency and the non judgments upwards frequency, the version of sustain evolution towards a path of elevation.

The challenge that many researches the experience is the field that adapt new methods (pos and cons) towards readapting and reconnect the individual with nature.

The modern technology separates natural law of the individual and law of nature as the appreciation and importantly reduce ways to elevate frequency within body positively.

The path of virtues and appreciation is a path that confront every human being at some point of living the elevation frequency as the important existence on the earth, life essence, humanity and eventually embrace or denies the free will, anyone can heal if they can believe.

The consciously or unconscious experience what makes life worth ticks as body and mind measures the ability to make the space and time connected as the individual differentiate the approach when crosses time on the earth.

The competition comes from different genes sharing different operations "individually" this challenge ables the improvement as the energy on the matter, the individual easily attaches the gravitational field, the ego (defined by Sigmund Freud) remaining as the way to elevate frequency challenging downwards frequency, therefore the spiral of energy on the earth frequency reaches many levels of frequency, the ability to vibrate consciously through the vitality reshape the upward reality applying on individual field, realign the frequency with a healed tone that create a natural flow of elevated frequency, the collective healing amplify the magnitude within modern world, it is absolutely powerful the light frequency that vibrates on the earth through this millennium.

49

The ones that appreciate simple things in life finds the path of inner peace reaching longevity because the matching frequency well balance. From the healing perspective the place of equilibrium and magnitude must start within body.

Imagine the frequency of longevity on the personal that lacks financial abundance or a person with financial abundance that lacks a healthy life, the fulfillment of life comes from the present, measuring living upward frequency available and accessible through the natural healing operating within individual body and mind.

The appreciation of life on the earth, breathing, sharing the journey, the phases of life and self improvement as nature continues to be the main technology, the vibration of earth elements that the individual appreciate the natural gift and capability that ordinate, dominate, becoming present from the beginning to the end.

The energy is in constant change thus frequency matches beyond matter and the atomic elements creates the habitual frequency, life is the pulse that elevates and activates particles on the magnetic field attracting and synchronizing.

The individual beliefs is the abstract frequency between old and unprecedented believes the matching frequency becomes the pulse frequency that manifest everyday millions of life.

The competitiveness of the habits and habitat justify the attachment on the matter, exercise healthy habits program the mind to the appreciation of the habitat and others that are sharing the journey, practice rationally ways with nature and find the divine, the healing does not need to be a rocket science to experience as pure natural vitality.

We learn practices, dedication, teamwork that helps towards manifestation of the better frequency, by survive and revive, the action of the individual continues collectively healing , there's no better time than now to be selfless on the gravitational field and fully practice minimalism and embrace millennium ways to improve, be kind and communicate with nature.

* the Balance*

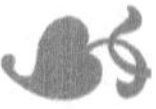

Be in control of two distinct elements, positive and negative reveal the atomic particles presented in nature, in the balance confront different living elements place order in the chaos and uplift energy. The living a life of uncertainty leads to self deprecation, self preservation comes from a life of certainty.

The chemistry balances the individual overall energy, when there's imbalance within body the vibration and strength decay, the balance and vitality relies on the frequency of the thrives frequency and holistically strengths the living essence.

The balance frequency reshape and tune through nature, vibrating through the air , sounds and particles. The balanced upwards frequency within mind and body unleash the motion.

 The elevation of the consciousness between reality and fiction leverage every fragment of reality, the individual thoughts are real for them and become the result belief of the frequency on the magnitude that evaluate thoughts frequency as ways to activate the upward frequency the alternative medicine methods creates balance on the mind, believing that the light (bright side of the mountain) or the darkness (the dark side of the mountain) when mind energy vibrates the body's energy integrating life as the process of evolution, factually the vibrational field of life is in constant motion.

The universe resonance compress body's frequency, resonating frequencies eg. (sleep and awake) vibration creates cycle, the individual conducts the matter through instincts, the mindset and the energetic balance within body.

The upward frequency creates viability channelling the universe (creator frequency) the return to the origin is the awaking inspiration continuously in creativity.

The combination of god's essence, infinity and balance, the real essence of existence lies on living elements between earth and spinning the frequency .

the language and gesture on every living element ticking
differently and dimensionally within space and time.
The impact of people's action and reaction , the solution is the
barrier that makes oblivious to the pain experience as the gravity
numbs the ability to heal, measure and balance this pain creates a
better the communication, acceptance of the process manifest
vitality towards the individual pursuit of life.
To create new possibilities, upwards frequency must elevate the
tone frequency present in nature, the universe and the collective
resplendence sounds creating meaningful vibrations and intention
of healthier living elements, the positive nourishment towards the
(thriving effect) the appreciation of the conscious of the individual
and the collectiveness of the individual.
The vital vibration within environment is the healthier favorable
communication that vibrates and balance (reflecting the state of
mind) works to the reverse cognitive dissonance and elevate self
improvement.
 Life frequency is a processual modus of vivendi, the mind of the
individual works through relatable frequencies, circumstances,
riddles and rising solutions accordingly with the elements of
attachment and its necessary methods that transform the energy ,
the landmark of consciousness and the awareness of the frequency
requires the equilibrium pulse.
The variability energy increase therefore through the application
of living the ethical life, one can request from an oblivious person
virtues without support the process of virtuosity, it will not happen
the modern world identify the importance of righteousness as a
shift of the reality, the truth is that the individual without
introduce basic respect for the nature cannot acquire frequency as
generated from the belief, the experience of living a healthier life
(modus vivendi) differentiate as a new creative era where the
individual access the well balance life experience and recognize the
ones within process of betterment and control frequency duality
and relies on the law of simplicity and reciprocity, the humble way
to balance the frequency.
The detachment process dealing with matter, identifying the
elements of duality, electrons, protons, ying , yang, feminine,
masculine,hot,cold and overall dual synchronicity .

The embracing of duality helps to identify the better way to elevate the frequency. The modern time to recreate the conscious upward frequency, eliminating negative thoughts, old beliefs, cognitive resonance, exercising the natural phenomena swinging through the frequency, practicing a new and better way to improve towards healthy lifestyle with alternative methods can be manifested the present reality.

Chapter 05

Time and Reality

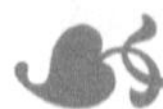

What the law of relativity means nowadays to the modern world? Time is the effect of life as energy creates movement, time remains the unsteady force of the abstract field recording, evolving and connect with gravity through cycles and measurements.

All living particle moves its own finality (reality)

The fragment of time is relative, element's variates time as existence and adaptation.

The habitat attaches the magnetic field, time is the fragment that contributes to the overall reality, fractions between space and time that can makes two segments distinctly on the mind and the body obliviousness, if you ever heard concepts of time such as (You only live once, You only have this moment, living todays there's no tomorrow...) time sets many to fail, time happens accordingly with life, many acquire time differently on their own frequency of life. The solution to recreate time, reverse primitive nature i the progress, self transformation and relatively uplifting frequency as apply genuinely the law of proactiveness, manifesting of the environment, collectivity to another person, daily and without exceptions of classes, race and opinions as result when applied genuinely proactive turns nature's frequency into the meaningful reality.

A second*

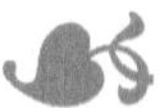

The universe will give you what you deserve? that's not really true. The universe gives time abundantly and based on the integration the individual relationship with time and preservation creates capabilities that evolve and growth and connect with fulfillment. The awareness of the moment is the creation presented now. The one must become a protagonist of the life and scale to the leverage and improvement.

The world continues delivering the same frame, nothing really changed from the operation level, what opera thought us about comedy and tragedy, villains and hero, innocence, queens, kings, the fool and the archetypes. These characters plays the environment that surround each of us aiming the elevation of the moment.

The individual plays the environment every second, does you connect with your nature proactively? the collectiveness rises and brings the most important sequence of the divine essence.

To recreate time and manifest healing it is necessary to feel the connection with nature through the time, pulsing without waste the essence and recover steady with discipline.

To understand the healing principle time becomes the equation, (adapt, add or subtract) to heal eliminate time, (the old patterns), time is the technology that many individual thrives to create the real experience (addition or reduction) easy equation (time - environment + you = -x) or the equation of productivity (+time+environment+ you = +x) find your X factor with time and space. The second creates values, the time does not exist unless fragments are real, the second of time (intentions) breaks old patterns and primitive nature, the genuine cycle of time is the environment shapes of frequency, the free will endure time.

Time makes the world ticks as the offspring makes time ticks, the relationship with time is reciprocity and synchronicity complement every second, minutes and hours.

The alternative medicine supports the thriving process as time
manifest a healthier body, mind and soul. The longevity through
nature repaired with the frequency, methods as equation towards
the balanced life.
Every second emotions and motion consciously and unconsciously
thrives manifesting nature's growth.

Accuracy *

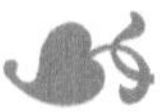

Time accuracy and the infinite equation, the repentance of cycle spins building through breaks and decisions. the free will of each individual define their time and the evolutional process of each individual is the embrace of its way of life and the will forward to the essence.

To better understand time accuracy practice the gardening, the bean can have an accurate seven days to sprout, nature is precise. The life is a experience that must blooming through time, it does bring cycle of evolution.

The perception and the mind focus eloquently as the result of the matter, time travels in waves and manifestation.

To begin a healing process there must be a commitment with time, set the time to recreate and affirm the release of old patterns and activate the vital connection with nature, the time well invested increase longevity, it build new experience nourishing the essence between the abstract world, the origin, body essence, mind essence and soul essence (Chi) that concretes the time essence. It become interconnect with the environment reviving the relationship with the matter between time appreciation and transmuting the depreciation with cycles of nature and its season towards a healthier lifestyle. The conscious ways to absorb and manifest activate time and space, the unconscious time, introduce relative way to interact with the essence and the field of perception.

The perception of self and others outside of ourselves, genetically mates attracts probabilities to recreate a better way of breakthrough the downwards frequency, engage in relationships is the connection with frequency, the balance and harmony through time.

To balance time and space practicing virtues is a conscious way to experience quality of life, time and reciprocity and recognize the neutralized scale point, revitalizing the present time, breaking up old patterns and expand the healing path through decluttering and proactiveness.

protagonist thrives within essence, antagonists thrives in destroy the essence, what makes life ticks? Balance life to the conscious harmony, applying facts, and recognize the effort the individuals places towards their own pure healing alternative holistic essence. The importance of healing the body activates the renew process as the awareness of the moment within body, therefore many holistic methods support the body such as sauna, baths, water cleansing, clear mind and the support the stimulation of new cells.
The commitment of renewing and rejuvenate through alternative medicines requires the individual to set the time cleansing the body, go to bed at certain hour and wake up on time, create new habits that support the individual body, mind and soul reset.
The time essence revitalizes, the importance to accept the creative method and elevates the essence of the body continue practicing self love and nature hold us dearly, the nature response on the absorption of the present time, valuing the moment, healing the individual of unnecessary emotions, effectively rising the realization of time, increasing positive flows within cellular level, activating time and complete levels of emotions, productive is realize time and recreate ways to apply effective methods

Chapter 6

The individual universe

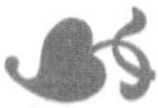

To know "thyself"in such genuine way of fulfillment and to balance the emotion with the relationship with nature (motion) allowing a healthier lifestyle therefore respecting the universe of others.

The awareness of your universe is crucial to find constructive ways to experience vitality and reverse self sabotage and self absorbed mindset but revealing the unique inner individual universe, breaking downward frequency to balance the way, positively, be aware of concrete and abstract ways to elevate the essence.

The universe script life repeatedly project "Self" the modern world that made easier for recreate ways that understand likes and dislikes of the individual's universe and the frame that contributes to the manifestations proceedings, recognitions, excitement and end (Life and Death).

To create and define the essence of a healthier life, first accept that everything is naturally in synchronicity and on the right place vibrate space, change the structure with the time, it depend on your abilities to renew the process and must embrace the universe law of acceptance and the nature of self.

 The universe updates intentions and manifestation the reality on elevated level, therefore independently thoughts are the universe channel between the individual's universe, choices and free will manifested in the field.

*Cause and Effect *

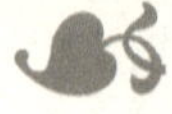

The individual is the cause and the effect.
The cooping effects are self sabotage emotions, the emotions
evolve as old patterns thus remaining consciously attached to
relief emotion. The cycle of motion working on the effect of the
particular frequency, it can be reversed as any individual can
break unhealthy lifestyle cycles on the frequency of recognize the
emotion and accept changes on the pattern shifting and reconnect
(cause and effect) in order to recreate an elevated frequency,
therefore the individual must within vessel (body) release
judgments (broken frequency) operate on the highest frequency of
healing (transformation) the universe is a constant vibration
moving of the effect.
The first experience of a new born with the gravity is the contact
with its own emotion, life sensory is activated on the emotion
shifting the gravitational field, the gravity density impacts energy
therefore rising the effect of the frequency, manifest emotion is
within core of every being alive.
The practice of meditation helps to manifest, shifting and
reconnect repairing life adapting new habits and beliefs that
reduce emotion from pain to overjoy balancing emotion with
motion, accelerating vital vibration with mantras to connect with a
healthy relationship with self.
The healing begins when the individual addresses gravity in such
healthy way refuse living the effect but create through time (begin,
middle cycle and the end) the positive cause.
The individual's universe must respect the primary law of nature,
the provision, breakthrough victimization and embrace cause and
effect. The practice of natural healing helps to connects with the
living effect regenerating naturally with the universe of the
individual vibrating through motion and emotion, perceiving as
neurotransmitter processing body chemistry balancing the
individual's universe vibrating cause and effect on the healthier
pursuit of life.

The mindset frequency connects beyond time as the ether synchronize with the transformation of the individual from the unhealthy habits towards a healthy universe, granting this important process to embrace holistically and naturally achieving a vital, healthier lifestyle.

Individual's universe consciousness *

The chemical elements present in the habitat becomes the overall oxygen of the particular individual, therefore chemistry effect such elevates or decrease consciousness changing or unchanging the gravity field creating necessary pain (unhealthy cycle) completing the expand and elevated consciousness.

The rationality of the individual guides the way towards the element, manifesting beliefs and improve the way to communicate with the universe.

The essence and absence is the modification through the constant evolutionary process vitalize the essence operating on the higher frequency level, exercising life, essence and dimension therefore the provision must be appreciated, the emotion of acceptance creates the energetic frequency on the field of accomplishment on ways that exercise the virtues and elevate manifesting the healthy frequency.

How to recognize time shifting frequency of life and healing. The mind recognize the message of the frequency as the universe tune on change.

The atomic structure, every single component of the individual reality reaches the intention purposely and elevate the individual, the frequency setting the produce and prioritize the fundaments of life and its experience, if the particular universe doubts the process the operation decay consciously because of the belief, everything or nothing is the improvement, observe the universe around as triggers the emotion and conduct towards the experiences on the daily embrace process as the life happens through the universes lenses.

The consciousness is the certainty that avoid the allusion, everything is where suppose to be each message does speak to you, every experience happens, every message makes consciously nothing or everything, it does happen otherwise create the essence.

The moment the universe creates and recreate, truth versions activates the deep sense of the present reality.

To breakthrough the rules of illusion, living the perfect modern world surrounded with realization thriving on the better version of beliefs as the universe proactively operates on the healthy structure and lifestyle.

The individual's universe is the conscious realization of time, vibrating right through in alignment, the reveal compare and practice the gesture of balance in the chaos, the time remain ancient world to the millennium, many individual universe proved effective Earth is a place to heal body, mind and soul, the collectively everyone has been on the gravitational field as long extended and experience injuries, unbalanced as become oblivious of the structure, regardless of the universe hidden purpose as black holes, the time to rebuild, recreate, renew and reconstruct the elements activating the living purpose happens in synchronicity and pulse, as the universe is the now neutral point and does not contribute to the surround unless the energetic field is manifesting vibration, the individual contributes to the evolutional energy through the obliviousness, the capability of the individual to transform the universe consciously on the energetic field vibrating positively around is absolutely transformational.

What is the conscious better version of the individual universe? Is the genuine breakthrough of ego, selfishness, breakthrough fear, breakthrough trauma, breakthrough the conformism and release to the healing journey with a open mind and heart operating through recreate a better life, deeply decluttering, scrutinize actions and reactions and operates on the vibrational frequency of the proactiveness, opening the curtains and sight the authentic and creative shakes the structure.

To recognize and scrutinize the inner universe towards change, allows happens as motivates creating new habits without seeking rewards, practice change without expect but let nature motivates the way, the singular is the most important element of nature.

when the practice of elevation is activated, the most beneficial way
of change is activated, continue dreaming or awake the healing
reality to the healthier way of living.
To practice nature activating the cells particles as the atom having
positive and negative, making the right cooperative responsible
action, the introduce of the respect of the space, make it right to
recognize and avoid mistake emotion and the motion of the
moment, nature control on the superior, revealing the place to
heal. Practice consciously righteousness changes the frame of
mind, connects the environment energy thrive and recognize the
common sense, the continue healing manifest, recreate on the
discipline of peace, self awareness and the constructive part of the
Anima, the goal is to increase the awareness of the conscious doing
individually always distinctively proactive with others universe, as
the communication of others are in the level of reciprocity,
people's perception of life is individually, rationalize differently
and uniquely practice new ways to improve the self consciousness
without expectation compose the right inner universe structure
(anima) one cannot support the universe laws without evolve
through balancing ego, elevating the structure, accordingly with
the universe, unfold levels of manifestation as consciously
happening and unfold the different universes.
The individual's consciousness manifests the universe by practice
the break of old habits throughout predominantly creates
principles that balance the universes prioritizing the law of nature,
respecting human nature bio (life) as the individual life
experiences evolve beyond deathly matter continuously healing
alive and integrated with the world practicing the essence, thriving
healing self and respect on the way.

Chapter 07

The Universe

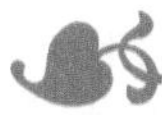

Does the universe conspire?
Yes, the universe actively spiral on the space as time spin trough the gravitational field, the universe matches frequencies with action and reaction nature.
The individual's mind, intuition and beliefs manifest actively in the constant and relative shift as the evolution occurs through the connection of the universe allows mind and body of the believer balance abstract and concrete life and ways of living.
The universe manifest healing within body, mind and soul through stages in the physical as implement the beliefs and manifest life.
The interaction with the universe is present within effect of the frequency.
The universe is conscious as synchronize the negative and positive vibration polarities, external and internal of the receiver (the individual) vibrate the belief, nature and environment frequency.
The universe give and receive on the frequency, the individual is a synchronicity sequence of X and Y chromosomes life.

* The language of the universe *

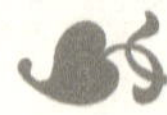

The resonance is the universe language and dynamics and magnetism is the force.
The perception on the theory of the gravitational field, focus on the receiver, explains the energy field of vibrations and the most important part of the dynamics the shift towards the frequency of upward spirals and the individual's manifestation.
The universe divide, adapts, align and re-adapt .
The defined growth on the living frequency elevating towards different polarities of the environment shift, the receiver and nature.
The language creates a pure genuine code, the individual achieve this language within their universe as a child and as adult through the decluttering process continue eliminate the human nature, pain, resentment, therefore the channel of pure frequency communication is a language that only the soul can be processed, beyond the matter the ascension of a pure state is the language of the universe, superior of feelings and experiences, the universe returns to the origin as a pure source.
The state of mind balancing the the individual communication with the universe language of virtues, the conduct communicates towards the tuned frequency.
Pure healing occurs when the individual allows the genuine connection within universe releasing the space of consciousness as the livelihood, essence and vitality within body, mind and soul vibrating the infinite state of blissfulness (Epiphany, shaktipa, nirvana, sheikinah)
The higher frequency of creation is the relationship between the individual's universe and the universes.

To apply healing, the pure intentions must be the elevation frequency manifested within space, the healing manifests through the balance of both frequency within body and complete the alignment of body, mind and soul. The universe, environment and mind creates the pseudoscience that reach epiphany.

The desire to control, entitlement, manifestation, and vibration of the frequency reveals the downwards cycle which through the process is the incomplete communication with the universe.

Two forces of energy operates within universe, times in balance and times outer balance, these constant shifts is the individual's connection with life, as the process rely from within consciousness, the individual finds levels of DNA imperfections as continue working on its own ways of ascension.

The frequency of the world is the matches magnetism in constant and continuously building the remaining process, elevating the frequency with nature, its the healing motivation towards the many ways of self improvement.

The universe inspire towards a better version of the individual, human nature can be upgraded, renewed and healed.

The operation of nature to break old patterns of mind and fully operates through cycles of life as the universe of the individual becomes aware of the unknown universe, the individual breakthrough and magnetizes constantly inside building continuous experience, many times thriving between healthy and unhealthy driving towards better result of manifestation as the individual dedicates to the process of healing with willingness, certainty and driving to the healthy universe manifesting the belief of the mind.

The Nature *

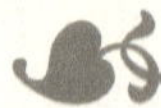

The human essence is nature, the roots of the DNA biological life components is the organic structure, the ancestry tree comes from nature, the human civilization acknowledges nature, even the scriptures acknowledge (you were made from dust) as the main foundation, the nature measures precise therefore nature compared with elements becomes the vehicle to thrive body, mind and ointment the soul. The laws of nature are clear of the synchronicity, therefore if the individual stops frustration but focus on Lear the laws, it precise elevate, balance and transform these laws, proven resourceful for the sake of wellbeing.
The nature of synchronization or desynchronization does not nullify free will, the main reason life is a brief experience on time is the improvement of nature on earth, the energetic field is the capable evolution of reality and time.
The healing manifestation through the universe occurs from the individual's desire as manifest and control.
The relationship with nature is the realization of the instinctual mind of the individual towards the universe as the synchronicity of the elements empty inside space of gravity adapting the importance of transformation.
The alternative healing allows the individual creates a higher consciousness allowing manifestation, readapt as the individual universe elevates a higher frequency, the space where body mind and soul frequency translate the pure essence of the universe.
The transformational process of healing and detoxification of unhealthy habits, first commit to the essence as the universe adjust and improve upon the individual's change, the power of breakthrough elevate new habits and laws that replace into the healthy acceptable way complete the healing operation.
The individual mindset continues manifest the frequency changing and unchanged as the same essence of the desire and willingness to continue the predominant magnet.

The nature is part of the universe practice as the universe channel the message of elevation, the nature shift the nirvana within body, mind and soul, the high consciousness when well embraced, old living habits are left behind as the living essence within universe pulses conspiring predominantly to the achievement of quality of life.

The composition of the universe relies on the habilitation and creation, therefore when the structure of the universe proactively achieve the level of consciousness elevating the synchronicity.

 Mastery the importance of universe shifts of time frequency of energy of life elevating from the zero scale towards life manifestation and breaking through the cycle of egocentrism and translate the shift of consciousness within overall body, mind and soul.

The nature essence is the chance throughout existence.

The universe thrives on the duality(yin and yang) as nature balance, the alternative balance of nature is the only way to elevate collective consciousness and support the balance of conscious and the unconscious.

The universe definition of infinity towards the way of living relies on the individual mind and the limitation of their way to integrate with nature, the essence of nature vibrates in superior nature elements supports the individual field on the frequency magnetizing different elements within matter, physical body composition and element.The individual destroy nature consciously or unconsciously as the body cells regenerate the composing element. It is the synapse within body a (fire), the hydrogen and oxygen (water) that transform oxygen (air) intoCO_2

The metamorphosis of the human body naturally connects with the element of the nature with humankind balance.

The universe magnetism into harmonious elements project individually and create life frequency, the vibration brings awareness of the upward frequency.

The foundation, principles and laws of the universe eloquently evolves within individual time and cycle of life.

The manifestation of the universe defined as the configuration of the nature as the individual through nature, identifying self frequency, shifts and send the message to the universe.

these frequency add towards different areas of life, as the modern manual to elevate soul constructively printed within nature and its virtues, respecting others within process of personal boundaries, elevating the quantify frequency ascension towards the collectiveness.

The nature prioritizes elements transforming life elevating, creating angles towards new perspective, continuing shift towards universe's elevation.

 Alternative healing is the best approach to support humankind towards achieve a healthier communication with the universe, channels of nature and manifest creativity, activates the awareness within body, brings discernment and vibrate the soul frequency towards a vital constructive life.

Life's essence makes the universe evolve and what creates a greater cooperation is the universe abundance, life within genes, healing and the pursuit of a balance the frequency of life.

* The Alternative Healing *

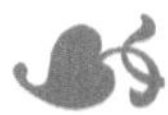

The nature synchronicity brings the importance of detoxification, the healing source within physical body releasing the external and internal unhealthy conscious and unconscious decision of the mind and soul. The body is the vehicle of the mind and soul through the alternated upwards and downwards frequency.
The elevation of the healing start in the cycle and daily healthy selection, morning through the night and the sleep cycle.
The body system function a healthy creative experience with the glands that supports the hormones, the mind and overall health. The basic experience of a better routine such as brush teeth with less chemicals, select an organic bath, detox periodically, be open towards healthy food selection to create better circulation, calm down nerve system activating parasympathetic through meditation (balance meridians) elevates the chakra supporting the healthy function of the organs, regulating digestive system detoxify from inorganic chemistry within body and accelerate the production of healthy hormones. There's many practices that support the healthier immune system, the process reverse diseases within cellular level, require healthy choices as new habits includes thoughts that helps the elevation of the body and mind, enhancing the performance of the physical body, producing positive results.
 The importance of healthy glands connects the body towards the absorption of mineral and vitamins, these nutrients supports the living particles as organic chemistry creates the vital force within body elevating towards a healthier physiology process supporting the genes of the individual..
The inorganic and organic chemistry is present within matter intersects the compounds as balance with nature, the goal is to reach resilience elevating the vitality within body, practices such energy flow as walking barefoot, feeling the grass, hiking, ocean bath, feeling one with nature embracing the healthy healing process reverse stress, trauma, injury and disorders, easily healing

the nature addressing precise diagnosis and prognosis of the individual and its vitality. The harmony and communication with nature is extremely effective for the individual, it does brings positive effects, stimulates healing, instincts, beliefs and mindset as well strength the genetics.

The healing essence and practices of new habits elevates the bound with the nature and its elements.

The practice of meditation (pray) toward the superior source of energy creating alliance with the (creator) God, Goddess, superior force, beyond the universe, the belief of the individual allied with the infinite giving source of life frequency, elevating sustenance channels and manifestation.The energy of appreciation and practice share with the universe channels giving and receiving , creating a timeline of healthy relationship with nature from the conscious level, as nature frequency gives endlessly, the individual frequency supports the process e.g (recycle and recreate)

The divine essence of infinite frequency elevates and control the nature prevailing over the technology, nature is the balance.

 The modern world of healing creates different technology that supports the energetic healing. recharging process of mind, body and soul, the resilience of the genetics through time, space and generation as the alternates perception of the individual works on the healing of the genetic organic structure, strengthening the performance towards acceleration of the time technology towards its accountability, communicating construction of artificial and reality adapting the modern society recreate the world reality

 The alternative healing is the breakthrough of the individual needs addressing health and exercise new healing methods to restore self and positive identity, the natural medicine addresses different feelings and emotions effectively releasing the somatic pain.

The levels of mind attachments holds body and soul, the natural healing is the methods that resets the unconscious patterns of the mind and recreate a conscious sight of life, reversing unhealthy decisions and the most important, working through self improvement.

The physical healing address different styles, emotional and mental applying the process of the body and mind aware of new tactics and consciously suiting to the interest of the individual.

The easiest way to experience healing is the understand of body, mind and soul livelihood, manifest the deeply evaluation, transforming the ordinary to the extraordinary, improving healthy lifestyle, contributing to a better experience of healthier life.
The priorities of the healthy life from toxic habits are replaced by the state of mindfulness, achieving the body and mindset of health. The important conduct vitamins, minerals and balance the chemistry aiming the individual wellbeing as the importance of continue the mindset training that access healthy consciousness and primarily begins the organic space where surrounds nature and embrace the environment, infusing the immune system healing with supportive nutrients fighting diseases create a healthy living.
Let thy food be the medicine(hypocrites) the fundamentals of healthy life relies on a body's nourishment and nutrients, by supports the healthy function of the body and the healthy mind. The body nourishments back to the nature fruits, vegetables juices and teas that reverse the risk of chronic diseases as the unhealthy patterns increase poor circulation (low frequency) contributing to the stress hormone decreasing body's vitality, chemicals elements present within food such as high sodium, refined carbs, sugar reduce the natural cellular process level to its vitality within body.
Alternative healing has been proven effective preventive lifestyle, relies on natural and different organic ways to achieve longevity
 The easiest way to practice and embrace changes surrender and breakthrough old habits, fully accomplish the self healing and fully exercise the mind consciously aligning body awareness and the positive soulfulness energy.
The alignment of healthy state of mind guarantee overall feelings and healthier emotions such as happiness and fulfillment of the core through the wholistic experience.
The cure happens when acknowledgement deeply grasp on the individual body, mind and soul.
There's an emotional factor of the healing process through the consciousness as much as oblivious and numb the individual's reality appears, overcoming effectively these emotions through the method of catharsis, regenerates deeply the process of the mind and body and find ways to elevate the frequency within body through natural nutrition.

The healthy organic food introduce different cleansers, detox, plant base, sustainable, bio-organic the natural water PH, these alternatives practices increase longevity, as well combination of chemistry that balance the body, such as juicing and teas to support the body filtering as well the periodically fasting to restore the digestive, these methods maintain the body ability to be healthy, brings oxygen to the body through greens and rejuvenating healthy plant base, healthy eating habits.
To invite nature and be part of living life creates alternative healing lifestyle to create the experience of unique and supportive cells, on the overall physical body health, free of chemicals and recreated on sustainable levels.
Healing the physical with phytochemical accelerates the production of healthy cells, creates body's anti-corps, strengthens and elevate body longevity.
The relationship with yourself is the key to elevate a healthy environment, enhance the energy, have a better performance, elevates self esteem , spirituality, compassion and communication with element of nature connecting between the universe and the beliefs of body, mind and soul.
Applying a healthy way of living accelerates the constructive connection with the universe and uplift energy.

Chapter 08

The words

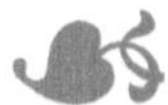

The ability to communicate is the most beautiful expression of life, words express the individual rationality, behind every DNA there's a trace of communication through body language, expression and gesture, the non verbal communication and the verbal communication, translate meaningful elements and sound truthfully rectifying and healing.

The primary concept of healing is recreate the ability to be understood, the healing occurs when there's a completion of emotion,physicality, psychologicandphysiologic,the feeling good effect and completion through the words and emotions.

The creative better communication helps the way of healing as the relationship with self reconnect.

The words vibrates and center the self, becoming the most beautiful symphony to the listener is the way mankind sound, it create a better expression through the words which have a power of elevation and destruction, beware of energy and the profound meaning of words spoken in the energetic field, the resonances results energies are magnetized in the concept of connection conscious and unconscious. The words throughout generations creates differences and similarities, the words result in control, resolve heals and create.

 The age of information played a major role, as the generation advances artificial intelligence, words of affirmation creates the bound of likability.

the healing process through the words releases somatic pain, the
methods of silence the mind and recreate words
 that manage deeply the frequency within energetic healing field,
the words reflection within body, mind and the soul.
The cycle of nature, the universe, the individual and the universe
of the individual connected by "words" receiving and giving
sounds of life and what makes the individual life pulse.

* The essence of words *

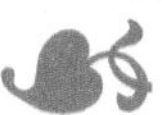

The essence resonates the energy through the frequency upwards and downwards, the alignment on the shift the frequency and balance the body, mind and soul, the essence creates a the wave vibration and the shift point on the process of healing.

The singular vibrates through the essence of its words, influencing the environment as the environment returns on the gravity control activating five senses, the nexus frequency vibrates the healing essence.

The speaking and listening synchronicity through receiving and giving frequency as the law of synchronicity elevates and differentiates unmatched vibration, the words on the frequency of the receiver creates the frequency that vibrates on the singular universe therefore the belief of the synchronicity manifests, the study on the field allows to appreciate matches frequency from the universe of the singular absorbed by different universe when allowed, through researches on the field of energy medicine the individual frequency can either cause the diseases as create the healing frequency.

The healing energy through words frequency balances and manage on the energetic balance upwards lifts reflects within mind and body.

The synchronicity creates the wellbeing towards healing as the messenger of the command on the synchronized frequency.

The message well communicated gratifies the listener reception, dealing with words, matching frequencies creates the elevation spiral of life, alternative healing on words frequency includes hypnosis, NLP,Mantras, Pray Pseudo approach on the communication.

The listener and speaker manifest life on the vibration of words, the importance to be present during communication is the human prints of evolution, the methods of communication recreate, matches frequency, procreates mates and agreements.

The communication brings life and capability of recovery as the art of ease, the words strength the immune system and heal.

Nature heals sending the words vibration to the receptor the frequency shifts. The words of frequency are affirmation and present in the habitat for the sake of the individual manifest as well gratify love, healing, elevation, blessings, fellowship, abundance and many other concept of positive communication enhance a greater lifestyle.

The giving is the universe sender practice and transforms the message to the individual into realization, the manifest channels creates through ease or disease frequency.

The communication credits the growing process as the elements of nature are ingredients of health as absorb the energy of body and mind, the communication is reabsorbed to the soul echos the magnitude of the frequency and each essence.

The spirituality is the language behind the frequency of the soul, elevating the frequency in many ways, words of life and virtues expand and define the lifespan , the pure healing frequency accesses a pure essence and energy.

The dosage of words elevate the mindset and amplify the constructive inner words of self energetically vital essence towards transformation and words that are the landmark of the singular, matching the communication and the commitment that evolve the elements.

To elevate healing within body speak words that elevate, match the frequency of words spoken and manifested as the single universe through universes cordially manifested.

 The sound of healing, connect with elements frequency, increase the tone and revitalize, the ether and the process on the oxygen manifests the vibration releasing the pain, recovery distress and reverse frequency elevating happiness, appreciation and redemption through the echo of the frequency.

Let the words speak through a healthy mindset, increase the wellness and the wellbeing of the mind, allowing the communication as the identification of the emotion, the language of truthfulness, virtues and individual consciousness is the language practiced towards change from psychology and physiology, the state of understand and living the balanced frequency as the universe identify on the sound of change.

The triggers of unhealthy lifestyle can be easily shifted towards healthy choices when triggers aren't oblivious or unknown but conscious to recreate choices as words activates the psychology and physiology on time of the singular universe brings the surface of the behavioral language and the mindset of the individual as the element surrounds the matter and the deep concepts translate half empty and half full on the belief of the individual.
The language of perception communicates the choices creating the reality.
The codification of a body, mind and soul reveals the full concept of the individual universe, nature and the frequency of the universe, identify as words that leads towards elevation and partially towards frequency where solution of the equation is the matched body, mind and soul frequency.
The body language and non verbal communication manifest the frequency, vibrating accordingly with the individual universe, this amplification attracts and repeal the absolute frequency, the matching frequency and synchronicity on the essence.

* Emotion and communication *

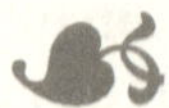

The individual adapts to the change through acceptance,
resilience, emotions and communication.
The frequency accelerates time spiring the individual between
universes and the recognition of the communication and body
magnetism.
The subconscious mind information concentrates the magnet
guiding the individual towards lifestyle that coordinates the
environment, beliefs, emotions, hereditarily beliefs, pursuit of life,
communication, biochemistry and between sympathetic and
parasympathetic responses of the nervous system the
communication increases the awareness of the body, therefore
memories of the body and mind releases subconscious expression
as the theory of mind specify the communication of the hidden
psychology of body language, the register of incomplete individual
emotion, nature and universe.
The nature of the individual register the message of somatic pain,
accumulating over the years within body.
the practice of Chinese medicine layout the meridians and the
elements of time to release the somatic pain within body, the
communication of body and mind have uniquely manner pulsing
the experience a complete vital universe embracing the duality and
the communication of the conscious mind.
The connection between human body, emotions and the influence
that resonates the mind on the alignment and equilibrium.
Life is the language of the soul, the element manifests different
emotions such as the frequency of elevation of the sphere of
happiness, joy and comfortable emotions.
 The individual perceive the message of life within DNA, the
translation of a life, translation of the soul cycle, the individual
interests, passions, hobbies, emotions, aptitudes, affinities,
communications, perceptions, identities, reactions, and ability to
create and destroy, all these records messages fulfills the
individual universe and continues the life experience as the words
assimilates the reached essence of health and healing pulsing life

vibration as additionally accelerates healthy feelings and lifestyle. The poorly communication raise the stress within body and raise the cortisol level on the abstract perception raising the inflammation within body and blocking the mind to absorb the message successfully, the mind understand the complete cycle of the somatic pain within body through a healthier communication a better frequency raised and healing manifesting the greater vibration.

The remedy of a healthy communication is recognize the miscommunication and develop the practice of receive the words as frequency in the level of re-create training the mind to register new ways to operate and amplify towards new possibilities for a healthy body and mind releasing records of resentments, fears and negative emotions shifting the cycle of somatic pain towards a pure healing frequency in the body on the shift scale of connect body, mind and vibrates soulfully.

The communication elevates the frequency managing the tone of vibrational frequency singing the bird melody on the healthy communication, many words spoken does not reach the pure state of transformation, the spiral of a grounded mindset dynamism the word training to manifest healing and guide towards consistency of a healthy life.

Chapter 09

Keys

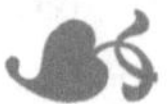

To create healthy decisions and heal the body through methods and abilities of doing so consciously, stepping towards a healthier vibration motivates towards unlock the virtuous keys of self consciousness of the singular mind relying on the healthier body, mind and the access of pure field of energetic cure through nature. The spoken words intents and desire speak the possibilities raises towards healthier healed life, the process of self awareness is the natural balanced emotions, the key of a healthy life is the embrace of preventive healing through nature and open emotion, the channels closing emotion, healing process of completion, longevity and renew of life.

The key of redemption surrender on the path of the recognized law of nature, the solutions relies on embrace elevating, divine connection, source, duality (yin and yang), balance (masculine and femininity) releasing the attachments and respect of the environment, the practice of redemption opens the channels of higher frequency with nature cleaning the frequency from the dusty vibration.

   The separation of conscious and oblivious managing balance on the body and mind creates the awareness of healthier life, the positive beliefs turns the key of awareness and support five senses, mind and body leveraging healthier experiences creating conscious choices.

The key is peruse and select your beliefs in such manner that elevates a healthy mind nourishing the essence of the body, understand the individual genetics type, spirituality is the ways to protect the overall body mind and soul on the perfect vital alliance of healthy way of living.
The conscious and unconscious experience towards a healthy lifestyle, guide the instincts of the constant changes and breakthrough old patterns guiding hereditarily way of health, making food priority decisions, reduce toxicity within body, allowing the nature connection on the roots and find group integration and prioritize a way of love yourself more, reviewing the keys and prioritizing moments of deep meditation and gratitude to ascension of nature within body, mind and soul. The natural practice that recreates the bound of the element health be present within nature.

* Unlock Body, Mind and Soul *

Imagine living the healthy lifestyle that pleasantly supports your own journey and consciously release the healing key of life.
 The compass for complete the essence of the being is the connection with the essence through materialize, visualize and make existent, through the colors matters create as the style shape and continue idealize and manifest the conscious feeling that connected with balanced belief that secure the vulnerable, the cause and the effect turn the key and release the mindset, lock and unlock as walk through the vibrational field of the transformational miracle tone and the willing energy to experience love unconditionally, accepting self love unconditionally as the healthy key for a better world.
 The unhealthy choices are the effect decisions made conscious or unconscious. The conscious creation of health are manifested on the gravitational field unveiling the unconditional self love practicing the universe life feeling deeply within soul, mind and body the key of thriving towards a healthier life.
The healing is the manifestation attained continuously as practicing fulfillment within heart and mind of the individual, be alive is the essence of the matter. The practice of natural healing unlocks the unhealthy choices and creates a healthy relation with the individual's universe, space and time.
The infinite light irradiates towards the consistent direction to achieve life and let the sequence of manifestation be superior of the circumstance, vibrating and channeling the remaining reality shifting point towards the healthy conscious life.
The livelihood of miracles happens where you can feel and experience the healing nirvana as unlock and create alternative healthy ways to the healthy connected evolved ways manifested consistently habitually.

The remedy to the unconscious is adapt the rational healthy life opening towards experiences nature creating consciously the stop and flow of the body, mind and soul towards the experience that breaks the superficiality, the numbness and the obliviousness allowing master within body and vibrates the healthy reality.
The door of the universe towards a conscious living must be unlock to walk the road of conscious emotions and introduce new methods of beliefs as recreate a balanced and thriving way from the gracefully appreciation scale vibration.
To release ego and negative beliefs knowing the key to open the door, the solution for the problem and resolve with self, resolution is the key that leverage experience on the overall completeness process of healing
The settings of wellness must separate, recreated and effectively heal towards the sharing and appreciation reality of the unique self, feeling completely comfortable with being.
The connection captivate and vibrate the essence towards nirvana of pure healing energy, pure healing consciousness and pure healing vitality.
 The self improvement is the key to access the nirvana state of healing relying on the willingness of the singular to create healthier choices as walking the road of healing and define the epiphany. The elements that supra-exceed the reality towards creating the fragment of a whole to connect the reality beyond the tuned healthier lifestyle.

* Living Soulfully *

What is the missed component for living a soulfully experience?
Feelings of acceptance, correction, completion and appreciation,
yet the most important is the understanding of the individual
healing process.
To elevate the essence it is necessary the fully engagement that
connect beyond the emotions but eloquently vibrates the
consciousness on the soul level towards the healthier and happy
living, as well allowing the experience flow from the sincere true
vibration, pure healing is the nature channel through the essence
of life, the planet of existence.
The evolution of the soul relies on the essence of elevation and the
matching essence of life through aspects of plenitude, the vital
energy of transformation, happening the physical and the
spiritual connection of the particular one and their unique
connection, the universe vitality pulse body, mind and soul
vibrating the movement of the energy, moving the essence towards
frequencies, the universe is the total alignment of the essence
supporting the process of elevation on the rising frequency.
The time and life of the matching frequency shifts constantly as
the difference between reality and the universes, the individual
have the key that lock and unlock positive the energy, the
importance of the healthy ways that allows matching frequency of
positivity law of return for mind, body and soul regardless of the
environment. The turn thrive on the higher connection operating
the frequency of living a life soulfully becoming alive on the born
frequency.
The beautiful art of release unmatched frequency and tune
emotion within world where protagonist and villains are the
consciously playing the nature.

The healthy conscious decisions, be aware of release toxic attitudes that blocks healthy behavior, avoid impulses, unlock resentments, overcome fear and stress relief, through the emotional affect, unlock ways to release the healthy healed living on the frequency, the pulses of the conscious life through the matter.

The frequency become the untold story through the belief of the individual for its certainty, the journey ahead of the meditative states transform methods using elements of nature, repairing the old story within soul level starting the way forward with positive intention as reconnect the positive emotion such as feeling the essence of the soul,(the epiphany)

The goal is to increase affirmation frequency of the mind, exercises longevity as the golden key for the conscious life, the body and the conscious element vibration as the universe and the reality of the soul, matches frequency of appreciation independent of how others pursuit their way to manifest their frequency.

The time and the space is the law of nature working effectively as well the respect for the nature of the particular.

The opening the genuine frequency elevates in realms as the creation of the conscious source of energy as the potential magnitude of the soul.

The expression of life is the upward energy, the lack of the essence creates the downward energy this alignment balances transformational realms of the soul of the particular essence, bringing the energetic healing from the deep heart, mind and soul.

The awareness of the element releases the somatic energetic field of the particular and beyond of the physical energy functioning within matter on the energetic field.

The higher energy consciousness is the surrender genuine spiral on the Krishna (Christos) surrendering the beyond, resuscitating the quality of life and self improvement, the healed life travels to the nirvana of the natural healing consciousness, revealing the epiphany, the higher dimension, turning the key to open the elevation of the reality.

The magnetic frequency of the energetic field spiral must vibrate on the transformation upwards pure healing energy.

The life cycle recreates through the nirvana as the genuine way to accept and evolve beyond the death point through the appreciation.

The practice of nature throughout masters the duality as part of the whole complete higher vibration of consciously connected to the energetic field through the universe language developing the language that strength that uplifting frequency and the most important, the awareness, to be the universe through the fragment of the matter and reveals the fulfilling comprehensive manifestation as elevating the truth strength of body and mind resonating fragments and desire of action and reaction.

The oblivious mind release and unlocked to the unconscious feeling allowing body and mind to embrace pure healing where nature pulses towards life, connecting the energy in harmony with the wellbeing.

The body regulates hormone creating homeostasis, the nature contact and balances hormones healing body's energy and connects towards healthier natural healing as the contact with energy increases the frequency energy supports the pure source of frequency available within glands (chakras) as the universe connects with the fulfilling energetic field of body and mind.

The alternative healing is the major release of the element as the particle balances different stages of life and evolution of the life.

The nature transform the spirituality creates the door of the divine energy, the translation through the frequency connects through the feelings of positive mastery frequency.

The meditative practices rises consciousness, repair the DNA, healing on the frequency triggering the elevated energy balancing mind, body and soul creating healthy synchronicity.

The nature is the structure necessary to the process healing steps, the Structure of the molecule, DNA's vitality presents the reality of time and space.The journey of healing unlock the present living creating the present essence channeling the constant energy frequency, the key is become conscious and aware of self and where to develop towards a healthy lifestyle.

Chapter 10

The fellow journey

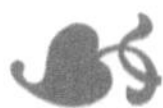

The journey intersect with elements that supports the healing
process embrace the benefits of nature to balanced wellbeing,
the arriving journey where you make peace with the self (ego),
let nature guide to balance of life through the physical elements.
The alternative medicine allows the creative state of healing
surface within body and mind embrace the modern world of
healing as earth (Gaia) reveal the living single particles on the
space and fully access the practice that matches the frequency.
The practice of mediation helps release the positive approach of
body chemistry within journey including the struggle of arrivals,
in conclusion through the understanding and acknowledgment of
match frequency with space becoming fully present with the
nature and matter.
The Healing essence grounds and support the individual nature
path as the healing have the art of release emotions positively firm
through high ties, flowing quietly as channeling flows from outside
and inside the matching frequency, assimilating the elements.
The sustainability on the essence conserve through the nature of
the singular as the appreciation of the elements stables the essence
and balance the flow.
 The nature operates the major compound through the healing
outcome and balance of water, air, earth and fire of its essence and
seasons matching the body mass and mind.

A friendly space starts within soul level as the outside world is the spiral growth manifesting particular healthy frequency elevating the control of body mind and soul and the vital pulses essence(chi) the universes living frequency of elevation of its own livelihood.

The Bound *

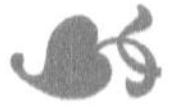

The universe resonates time, essences, path and interconnection.
The creation of upwards and downwards frequency is present
within individual and the journey, the effects, the strength and the
resilience of the mindset as energy motivates the individual and its
desire to overcome the emotion and motion reaction.
Recalling the emotions, desires, mind fragments, body physicality
and soul of the particular universe requires the transformation,
recreating and elevate the self love frequency.
The universe is created by indifferences therefore empty vessel
must prioritize attraction and flow from the zero scale creating
balance through a precise point towards elevating scale on the
reality of time and space between nothing at all and everything.
The distribution of different universes on the scale to manifest the
production of the reality and the matter, the world vibrates
through this stage and the key is withdraw healing from nature.
The healthy essence is the law of respect towards self, the family,
the neighbor and the living being, the contribution to the world is
become present through the simple gesture of genuine essence
manifesting within matter bounding constructively.
The principle of the innocence, recognize the path reflects the
choices and guide individual bound and protect the inner child.
The action and reaction energy inject focus moving outside,
growth breakthrough objects of attachment feeling the amicability
of the essence integrating throughout cycles producing
attachments and detachment of the outside world bounding in
synchronicity focusing within priority towards healing.
 Healing the particular time needed to the start point, creating
methods consistently as quality of life, exercise vitality releasing
them experience of now a positive sound of the soul.

The balance energy on the earth focus perpendicular comparing the planets in different resonance and the most significant frequency of balance. The life bound with nature happens to benefit the particles equalizing the earth as the favorable universe of the living element, a tree, a flower, a bird etc.. the universes tunes on the duality continually ahead as the modern world society test balance the duality of(mode of vivendi.)
The navigation of the emotions between healing the ego practice the control of meditation and equilibrium of the universes.
The alternative medicine have better methods that improve the lifestyle of the individual supporting the embrace through breathing and realignment to find the turning point that manifest soulfully.
The receptiveness of life unlock the horizon of the creative journey around the world, as well keep alive the consciousness on the natural, the preventive healing continue rising as new generation addresses the ability to create the healthier experience considering the struggles and circumstances that affected the world health nowadays, on millions of body, mind and soul must be conscious of the practice of alternative medicine rescues this generation and the longevity tree of life.
The remedy is manifest a healthy and vital life beyond the simple nourish life with laugh, bounding and share mindfulness and soulfully and alternative medicine guide ahead the process positively.
The methods of cure through nature and the reliance on the overall biochemistry, between the individual connection is the phytochemical that bound nature to the element as elevates life.
The parallels essence beyond matter and the combination contrast to reverse the essence of the elements annulling charges of the molecule structure within body, reverse the cellular code of the genetics to a healthier life.
The systems of the universe, stars, solar, planetary reveals light to the nature, making nature the crucial core of earth and the gravitational bond of life to value time and the changing moment, towards indivisible abstract level, the synchronic unbreakable bound materialize and create changeable structure.

* The Cycle *

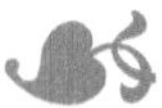

Earth cycle allows the continuous experience, as the integration with nature becomes the important relationship that exchange the epiphany of the soul, change the precise frequency of the particular time frequency of healing.

The elevation is the motion of a deep abstract level through the concrete field, the gravity exceed ways of living and motion towards the realms and find elevation on the purifying essence and recharge from the ill frequency throughout brings the nirvana in the motion that renew the essence of the energy cleansing the body, mind and soul.

The cycle is the dealings with the matter through downwards and upwards frequency is vital, the individual can mind its own elixir to the state of epiphany. The essence is reached with the assistance of nature, connecting the organs within body, screening the mind and elevating the soul magnitude through the miracle essence of the belief.

The manifestation of healing occurs when natures becomes the medicine, when the overall individual universe release in alignment the body, integrates the foundation the wholistic cycle. The level of body according with detoxification methods catalyses within cellular level, breakdown, cleanses and reverse diseases within the mind, body and soul, release a emotional response registered within soul through the cathartic process which is crucial to the individual that experience the category of healing.

 The nature is the balsam that operates chemically with nutrients activating healing as varieties of alternative methods within the essence of nourishment. The friendly vital force manifested within primal vitality (chi) strength, mastering this element through mindfulness, meditation and manifest the divine nature within individual universe.

The cycle of the frequency within nature includes creates experience reproduce through nature the greater essence in connection with the vital nature bond, it extend simple methods such as walking barefoot, eat clean, detox, stretching, breathing methods of elevation, amplify frequency allowing the growth of a healthy vitality, activating a strong level of consciousness and acceptance regenerating the cycle of the mind, body and soul on the earth.

Chapter 11

The story

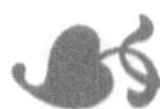

The extension of the individual essence through matched and unmatched roads of frequency as release the nature through the essential approach part of the process of life.

The applying process consciously reveal (cause and the effect)as energy growths significantly making life and the DNA level through the ordinary and extraordinary manifestation of the individual breakthrough, beyond the stop point of the frequency of the divine essence it becomes the part of the being alive

The universe travels time as years light creates heaven on the earth.

Say I am, to stimulate the vessel towards find the natural balance through herbs, sound and smell as open the earth gazes of organic transformations, none of the existing fact becomes important if the individual does not experience and practice the elevation of self with the pure heart.

The branch of the virtuosity is present within leaf along the road, walking on the earth road and continue release the memories within muscles, cells and DNA activating healing essence and growth through the process and the manifestation an appreciation of the structure.

* The dance *

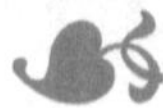

Every minute on the journey is meaningful and worth the
synchronicity.
Once upon a time bird sitting on the branch whispered the trails
road, looking into the eyes the bird sing these words.
Welcome to the forest where shifting starts, sharing the alignment
with the moon, stars and sun a sight, right there on the horizon,
releasing energetic healing as simple magical, beautiful and
sincere.
As the bid finished this sentence he flew away,
Would like to dance?
To Improve the healing experience, the willingness to dance
through the spiral where free will is activated.
This place of awareness from the simple living essence as the
flowers, the water, the day and the night creates the dances.
let the senses of the body aware as present become real, as we're
releasing the mind and reveal the power of synchronicity, dancing
with time as nature always on time.
The time of healing happens when deep affection gently touches
the pretentious veils between the untrue stories and the untold
stories. Healing is the true essence.
The stories that you will share with the world about your healing
will release the truth meaning of the dance, the song where there's
no misunderstood but the clear path of reached healing on the
sincere and virtuous release of the graceful vital essence of the
soul.
The nature recognize the living being and all the stories that
repeats daily, practicing the glorious moments as sharing the earth
kindly respect, shifting slowly dance gradual to the healing moves.
The recognition of healing from the consciousness through the
unconscious mind, reveal the oblivious emotion as address the
relationship with self, without sabotage the ability to be satisfied.
 Holistic healing helps the individual to find the inspiration to
write a new story of faith, many ways, even when your beliefs
didn't knew existed or possible as connect with the nature as fully.

The practice is remedy to elevate and balance the emotions as genuinely reconcile with the soul acceptance. Find the road where you can walk the recovery within accepting reaching the complete satisfaction as a dance.

The daily appreciation of living soulfully happy towards new possibilities, creates the road of appreciation compromise with self healing, Identify the body, mind and soul with thankful emotions creating the frequency needed to experience life coming from within body

The evolve of truthful feelings embrace moments as the result of manifest quality of life.

The restore of the inner self is present on the practice of acceptance, correction and closure towards an improved dimension.

To achieve freedom you can always appreciate the ones that conscious guide forward with respect, love and sincere sharing experience.

The truth essence of the spirit releases certainty the wholistic approach as eliminate self doubt filtering the pulse of life attracting the intense flow towards the spirit as essentially guide the road of sincere manifestation and genuine inner child ways to embrace give and receive life.

Alternative methods of healing helps to manifest and deal with balanced inner peace concentrating the creative ways that the mind of the achiever, heals through deep state of self improvement.

The healing integration is the overall health and wellbeing stage of advanced levels and the remedy of a healthy body mind and soul, regenerated constantly on the homeostasis and create a holistic way of vitality.

Bibliography

The research book relies on experiences and studies of the author Rusiane Almeida in the segment studies field and expertise alternative medicine and holistic healing.

The author had a fair contribution of different communities and support through the field of research. During alternative research expedition are exclusive from the author's work
This book has been made through extensive and the applied methods of alternative medicine,
There is factual documented of the author work and studies and among arts, sciences, universities, libraries museums and exclusive allowed for researchers in the segment of professional work and alternative medicine

About Author

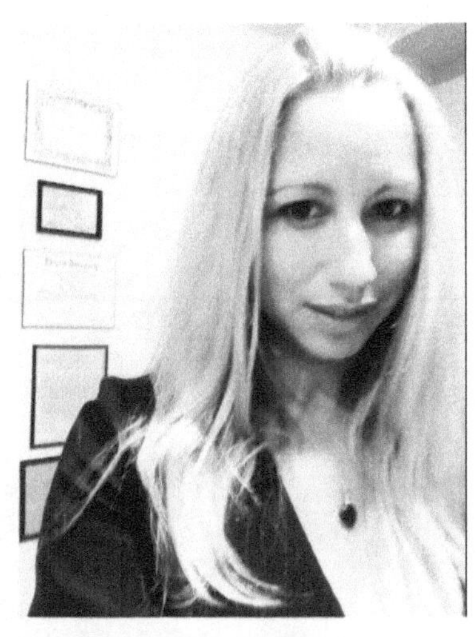 Rusiane Almeida study arts and sciences, originally from the Amazon Brazil rainforest where she resided until age of 17, her adopted father was a pioneer entrepreneur and founder of Amazonian village. Rusiane first journey abroad initiated her first business development project in south America, her passions includes languages, travels and explore new cultures, among her studies you can find law studies and fashion arts.

As young adult Rusiane Almeida moved abroad to the United States of America with her beloved family where she dedicated for project development, technology and the field of holistic healing, the author extended education for the bachelor in science in Alternative medicine, over the past seven years Rusiane Almeida worked in the holistic field licensed in different states as a therapist, Rusiane practiced therapies and help many individual healing and recovery methods included posture alignment body, healing and physical rehabilitation, Ms. Almeida projects includes Amazon Pure Healing the holistic therapeutic practices with her unique methods and healing approach.

The author writes about her field of expertise and inspired fictional stories as part of her hobbies , she advocates natural healing for body, mind and soul, she also travelled significantly executing her creative work, studying communities abroad , crafting and mastering her skills.

The author many work includes PR for non profits and private companies for the hospitality business and political activism pro community developments.

Index A-H

Index H-R

Index R-W